B-15: THE "MIRACLE VITAMIN"

B-15
THE
"MIRACLE
VITAMIN"

by Brenda Forman

Fred Jordan Books/Grosset & Dunlap

A FILMWAYS COMPANY

Publishers/New York

FRED JORDAN BOOKS/Grosset & Dunlap

Grosset & Dunlap, Inc.
51 Madison Avenue, New York, N.Y. 10010

1979 PRINTING

Printed in U.S.A.

Contents

1

What's All the Fuss About?

If somebody told you that there was a pill you could take that would give you more energy, improve your sex life, and cure you of some dread diseases, what would you say? That you'd try it and see what happened? That it couldn't possibly be true so it must be a hoax? Or that you'd play it safe and wait to see what happened to anybody else who tried it?

Well, those are exactly the claims that are variously being made for something called Vitamin B-15, a relatively new arrival on the health-and-nutrition scene. And depending on whom you ask, you can get any of those answers—plus others less printable. B-15's advocates (a group that includes many highly respected physicians) maintain that three to six of these little white tablets a day can have dramatic therapeutic results in conditions ranging all the way from ordinary fatigue through faulty sexual performance to serious illnesses such as diabetes, cardiovascular ailments, alcoholism, allergies, autism, and schizophrenia. Some even believe it can help treat or prevent cancer.

Needless to say, a lot of other people think that's all hogwash. The medical establishment, by and large, regards B-15 as a "hoax" and a "ripoff," unworthy of serious medical attention; the pharmaceutical industry doesn't think it's worth investigating; and the U.S. Food and Drug Administration hates it, maintaining that it's not a vitamin at all but a food additive and therefore subject to a lengthy list of restrictions on its sale and use. Maintaining that no adequate evidence has been adduced to support the claims its supporters make for its benefits, the FDA has forbidden research into the effects of B-15 on humans, has banned its sale in the past, and has on occasion confiscated shipments of it.

This in turn has elicited angry charges from B-15's supporters that the FDA is in cahoots with the medical establishment and the drug industry to protect their economic interests by keeping a substance with major curative and preventive potential away from the American public. Even several of the medical doctors interviewed for this book remarked that it was bound to get a lot of medical and pharmaceutical groups up tight if they thought there was a possibility that people might not necessarily get so sick so often.

All in all, it's quite a spirited clash, and it leaves a lot of people wondering just what the facts of the matter might be. Just what, in short, is all the fuss about? This book sets out for you the opinions and arguments on both sides, tells you about some of the intriguing evidence that has accumulated to suggest that B-15 may indeed have some remarkable possibilities, and discusses some of the questions that need to be investigated before the arguments can be laid to rest.

Where did it all get started? That's one of the first arguments you discover when you begin researching this subject. The most widespread account is that in 1951, a California biochemist, Dr. Ernest T. Krebs, Sr., and his son, Ernest T. Krebs, Jr., who specialized in treating illness through vitamin and nutrition therapy, isolated a crystalline substance from extracts of the kernels of apricot pits. Because they later found the same substance in the seeds of a variety of other plant life, the Krebses identified it generically as "pangamate" and described it, in accordance with its chemical properties, as "pangamic acid." Since pangamate was found in minute quantities in nature wherever the members of the B-Complex vitamins were found, and since it was the fifteenth such B-

Complex substance to be identified, the Krebses designated pangamate as Vitamin B-15. Still later, they reported that they had isolated the same substance from sources other than apricot and other plant seeds—from rice bran, brewer's yeast, steer blood, and horse livers, to name a few.

But FoodScience/Da Vinci Laboratories, currently the leading American manufacturer of B-15, vehemently contests this account. They maintain that for several years before the Krebses announced their discovery, the Japanese were working in the field and that in 1950, a year before the Krebses published their report, the Japanese had already isolated a new biologically active fraction from the liver and called it B-15. Even before that, in the late 1930's and early 1940's, they say, the Germans were working with a form of B-15 and noted its importance in internal cell metabolism.

Moreover, they continue, it's very hard to say just what it was that the Krebses actually *did* discover, because their original report on B-15 left so many questions unanswered about the substance's physical and chemical characteristics. "All sorts of things are left hanging," reports Dr. Roger Kendall, FoodScience/Da Vinci's chief biochemist. "In such a report you would ordinarily expect the author to report all the basic characteristics of the substance he is talking about. That means its melting point, its solubility in solvents, whether it's an acid or a base, its molecular weight or its chemical formula, its spectral characteristics, and its mass spectral and chromatography data. Most of this is left unanswered in the original Krebs paper—and he hasn't published anything more on it since 1951!"

FoodScience/Da Vinci Laboratories believes that its own research has ascertained the specific composition of B-15, and furthermore, they insist, it is not a vitamin at all, but instead a "non-fuel nutrient," essential to cell chemistry.

This, it turns out, is a crucial issue in the B-15 controversy. Although when the Krebses reported their discovery, they called the substance they had found "Vitamin B-15," they never went on to establish the need for this substance in human nutrition, an omission that continues to plague the B-15 cause because, under United States law, nothing may be called a "vitamin" if no nutritional need for it has been determined. The way one establishes a need for a vitamin is to identify deficiency diseases that are caused by its absence. For example, a serious deficiency or lack in Vitamin A usually causes optical diseases, among others; scurvy is what one gets when chronically lacking in Vitamin C; the absence of Vitamin D can bring on rickets and other bone disease. But neither the Krebses nor anybody else has done this for B-15, and so the FDA says it cannot be a vitamin. If it's not a vitamin, says the FDA, then it must be a food additive; and that means not only that its supporters must prove that it is non-toxic, but also that it cannot be sold as having any therapeutic value without getting clearance from the FDA as a drug, which requires extensive clinical proof.

Wrong, says FoodScience/Da Vinci Labs, it's *neither* a vitamin *nor* an additive, but a *nutrient*. One kind of nutrient is the "fuel nutrient." Fuel nutrients are carbohydrates, fats, and proteins. They are called "fuel" nutrients because they supply energy to the body for all its needs. "Non-fuel" nutrients are substances such as vitamins and minerals that the body needs in small amounts, and which it uses along with other internal chemical reactions, but which it doesn't use for energy. This, they say, is what B-15 really is; therefore, the dispute with the FDA has been largely misdirected because it has focused on the burning issue of whether or not B-15 is a "vitamin," and that is completely beside the point.

Whatever the truth of this dispute, and whatever the truth of B-15's initial discovery, its subsequent history has been stormy. The Krebses were convinced on the basis of animal experiments and tissue-culture studies using B-15 that the substance had a property of extraordinary promise: it could feed more oxygen into body cells and tissues than ordinarily occurs there, and it could also increase the volume of oxygen that normally runs through an individual's bloodstream. If this is so, then B-15's possibilities are certainly phenomenal—because if you can increase the oxygen available to body cells, you can in theory cure or counteract all sorts of disease and degeneration. It has long been known that poor blood and cell oxidation are a primary cause of degenerative disease, accelerated aging, and, eventually, death. In pangamic acid, the Krebses felt they had discovered a substance that would stem the course of hypoxia—that condition in humans in which depleted oxygen supply causes the body's healthy cells to degenerate into unhealthy and disease-prone ones. If, indeed, pangamic acid restored or sustained the correct oxygen balance in the body's organic cell system, the Krebses hypothesized, many medical marvels were possible as a result. If most degenerative diseases came about because of a breakdown in the body's cell system, the discovery of pangamate was truly a miracle.

But when the Krebses presented their initial findings to several medical-research societies and government-funding agencies, they encountered only skepticism and indifference. The medical establishment roundly rejected it. American medicine has long been notorious for its hostility to the notion that proper nutrition can be a powerful means of disease prevention as well as a major therapeutic tool in the treatment of illness. The medical establishment still tends to choke on that concept, although things are beginning to change a bit of late. Twenty-five years ago, however, the hostility was unalloyed.

The government was equally unwelcoming. The U.S. Food and Drug Administration refused to accept the Krebses' designation of pangamate as a vitamin—and still does— claiming that the Krebses could not show that the absence or deficiency of B-15 in the human system caused disease. Moreover, the FDA maintained that the Krebses were unable to demonstrate either clinically or chemically how B-15 did what they claimed it did, namely, how the substance increased blood oxidation and promoted the "uptake" of oxygen into the cells and tissues of the human body.

Finally, since pangamic acid was extracted in its purest form from the kernels of apricot pits, and since apricot pits were known to yield high concentrations of natural cyanide—a poison—wouldn't regular ingestion by humans of pangamic acid promote a toxic side effect, destroying cells and tissues rather than rejuvenating them? Despite the Krebses' appeal that their findings warranted further research into the effects of pangamic acid on humans, the FDA remained unimpressed and forbade Krebs to engage in such experiments. And there, for a time, the matter rested.

In early 1955, Vitamin B-15 (or pangamic acid) appeared on the European market under a variety of brand names. During the years that followed, it became widely used on the Continent and gained a large following, getting headlines as the "Doctor's New Weapon." As the years passed, at least ten other countries, including France, Germany, Italy, Portugal, the U.S.S.R., and Spain, have contributed extensive literature on it. But it remained relatively unknown and unused in America.

Then, in the early 1960's, a train of events began that was to give B-15 a new and powerful impetus in the United States. It involved the personal drama of a wealthy American family and yet another controversial substance also discovered by Ernest Krebs: Laetrile. It also brought a major new player onto the scene: the Soviet Union.

Laetrile was also first extracted—by Ernest Krebs—from apricot pits. Krebs labeled it Vitamin B-17; and from its beginnings right up to the present day, it has been a subject of passionate controversy between those who see it as a golden promise in cancer therapy and those who are convinced it is a specimen of dangerous pseudo-science. Be that as it may, in the early 1960's, a wealthy Italian-American family named Orlandi sought out Ernest Krebs when the elder Mrs. Orlandi developed breast tumors that her doctors felt could turn cancerous, especially since she was extremely tumor-prone and had already had four other breast surgeries. The Orlandis' doctors had recommended a double radical mastectomy. Needless to say, Mrs. Orlandi was distraught. The Orlandis decided to try Laetrile therapy instead. Krebs secretly administered his B-17 therapy to Mrs. Orlandi, and, within two weeks, the tumors disappeared. The Orlandis were convinced that Laetrile had indeed accomplished the cure and were so grateful that they offered to support Krebs' Laetrile research. They invested several million dollars into a Canadian company named Biozymes International, Ltd., that had purchased Krebs' patents to the manufacture of Laetrile, and, as an afterthought, to pangamic acid—B-15—as well.

Biozymes International did not do well in Canada, however. It ran into the same sort of opposition on the part of the Canadian government—which tended to take its lead in such matters from the U.S. Food and Drug Administration—that the Krebses had earlier encountered from the FDA itself. Intense lobbying of the Canadian government on the part of the Orlandis' partner in Biozymes, Andrew McNaughton, was to no avail. Moreover, relations were deteriorating between the Orlandis on the one hand and McNaughton and Krebs on the other, because the Orlandis believed that McNaughton was stealing their money. They decided to develop their own research into Laetrile and pangamic acid, and formed their own companies—FoodScience for the health food trade and Da Vinci Laboratories for the medical profession—to manufacture pangamate in tablet form. Ernest Krebs, Jr. (Ernest Krebs, Sr., has since died) and the Orlandis remain on less than cordial terms to this day, with Krebs indeed waxing vituperative on the subject.

While all this was going on, the Russians began getting interested in the Krebses' initial report on B-15. It is an intriguing aspect of Soviet science that whereas freedom of inquiry can at times be brutally suppressed in some areas where the authorities fear its findings will conflict with Marxist ideology, it is more daring than ours in others. For example, the science of genetics was set back decades in the Soviet Union when Stalin declared Lysenko's theory of the transmission of acquired characteristics to be state dogma, and sociology is still sternly constrained by the State authorities who are more interested in how Socialist Man *ought* to behave than in how he acually does. Yet it was the Soviets, not the Americans, who first ventured into space, and who are now reported to be conducting serious research into psi abilities and extrasensory perception. Similarly, it was the Russians who decided to explore the potential of B-15. They picked up Krebs' old patent on pangamic acid, altered the chemical formulation of the substance in accordance with their own experimental work, and filed a new patent—in the United States—on their own version, calcium pangamate. Subsequently, when Dom Orlandi saw this version of B-15 on display at Expo 67, he became convinced that his erstwhile partner, McNaughton, had sold the Biozymes formula to the Soviets. Ernest Krebs said he gave it to the Soviets. One more item of controversy in what is already a crowded field.

But the Soviets did what FDA hostility had made it impossible to do in the United States: they began studying the effects of B-15 on human beings. The results of these studies have been both the blessing and the bane of the B-15 cause ever since. On the one hand, they constitute the only significant existing body of serious clinical research to date into B-15's effects on disease. On the other hand, they leave a lot of critical questions unanswered because of what the American biomedical community regards as their sloppy and casual research design.

But the Soviet studies, whatever their shortcomings, are not to be dismissed lightly, for they constitute a startling compendium of provocative evidence, all pointing to the conclusion that B-15 has astonishing therapeutic and curative properties. Even an FDA assistant associate director for nutrition and consumer science admitted as much back in April 1978, saying that he'd read the available literature and that "the Russians can't be all wrong." The Soviet effort, headed by Doctors Yakov Shpirt and Yuri Udalov, used B-15 in the treatment of an exceptionally wide range of conditions, including such diverse illnesses as oxygen starvation (hypoxia), alcoholism, mental retardation, diabetes, gangrene, cirrhosis of the liver, and cardiovascular ailments. Their first group of reports was made public in 1964. They were very dramatic. In essentially every condition tested, the Soviets reported that pangamic acid produced favorable results.

The Soviets were especially impressed with B-15's beneficial effects in treating "cardiovascular disorders associated with insufficiency of oxidative metabolism," and considered this to be pangamic acid's principal field of application. Working with elderly heart patients at several hospitals in Moscow, the Russians had proved to their satisfaction that B-15 in the form of calcium pangamate is indeed effective in alleviating symptoms of arterial sclerosis. One hundred and eighteen patients, all over 50 years of age and suffering from coronary sclerosis, were observed after being treated with calcium pangamate. Both subjective symptoms (headaches, chest pains, shortness of breath, and so on) and objective characteristics (blood analysis, electrocardiograph findings, etc.) were measured on a before-and-after basis. Startlingly good results were obtained in 49 of the cases, with most or all symptoms completely disappearing and the patients returning to apparently normal health. Satisfactory results—a measurable lessening of symptoms—were obtained in 55 cases.

Even if this had been all, the Soviet studies would still have been worthy of consideration, since heart disease is the ranking killer in our society and any seemingly effective therapy should be worthy of closer investigation. But heart ailments were only the beginning. Shpirt and his colleagues applied B-15 therapy to several other diseases, including alcoholism, sclerosis of the liver, cardiopulmonary insufficiency, atherosclerosis (hardening of the interior cellular lining of the arteries), and diabetes mellitus. In each instance, the results were similarly favorable. The diabetes mellitus reports are particularly arresting. In many instances, reported Shpirt, calcium pangamate arrested the inevitable gangrene and forestalled amputation of the lower extremities, and at the same time brought about a reduction in blood sugar and sugar excretion in the urine. In mild diabetics, the administration of calcium pangamate "reduced the blood sugar to the normal level with simultaneous disappearance of sugar from the urine, thus confirming the assumption of the stimulating role of calcium pangamate in glucose oxidation." Concluded Shpirt: "We established for the first time clinically the therapeutic effect of pangamate in diabetes mellitus."

Some of the case histories indeed read like miracle stories. The feet of one man were literally rotting away with gangrene that had not yielded to any previous treatment. His doctors had given up and were recommending amputation. Yet calcium pangamate, according to the Soviet report, not only halted the progress of the gangrene but caused the sores to heal. In the end, the man could walk again. Whatever faults one may find with the Soviets' experimental techniques, notably their typical omission of a control group, this sort of report certainly demands closer attention. It's hard not to feel that we owe it to ourselves to find out just how much there is to this story. It would be so tragic if it were true—even if only in part—and we failed to follow it up.

The dramatic Soviet findings seem to support one of the major claims of B-15's supporters as to its biochemical behavior, namely, that it increases the volume of oxygen in the bloodstream, thereby promoting more efficient cleansing of disease-inducing toxins from the body's organic system. Like Ernest Krebs, the Soviets were unable to explain definitively just *how* pangamic acid did what it did, but they were sure that it *did* produce results. "Although we still do not know the biochemical mechanism of pangamate," wrote Shpirt, "we do know from our findings that it has a definite therapeutic result in well over 80 percent of the cases of each disease we have applied it to. It is safe to postulate that the original claims made for it by Krebs et al. are true, and that through the phenomenon of oxidation intensification, it has the capability of delaying or retarding natural cellular aging, the prime culprit in degenerative disease."

That same year, 1964, addressing the Institute of Biochemistry of the Soviet Academy of Sciences on the treatment of aging and senility caused by hardening of the arteries that feed and oxygenate the brain and other vital organs, Dr. Shpirt concluded his address by saying, "I believe that the time will come when there will be calcium pangamate on the table of every family with people past forty."[1]

If the Soviet reports of B-15's oxygenating properties were substantiated by other research, the implications for medical science would be earthshaking, because oxygen and its flow within the body are pivotal in the maintenance of healthy cell chemistry. Any number of degenerative diseases are either caused or exacerbated by depleted oxygen supplies to the cells. Every vital organ in the body is made up of an intricate cellular structure, all of them dependent for their viability on oxygen nourishment. This nourishment is carried in the blood. But when the bloodstream and its associated organs (such as the heart, lungs, and kidneys) cannot produce enough oxygen, or when the cellular structures are unable to absorb what oxygen there is available to them in the bloodstream, they tend to seek other forms of nourishment from other chemical reactions available to them in the body. It is these substitute forms that transform healthy cells into cells prone to disease.

Indeed, this metabolic substitution may be at the root of cancer. Dr. Felix Warburg, a two-time Nobel Prize winner, has advanced a theory about cancer's origin that is gaining increasing attention and that raises important questions concerning our whole approach to cancer therapy, as well as pangamic acid's possible applications therein. "The primary cause of cancer," Warburg told a gathering of Nobel laureates in 1966, "is the replacement of the respiration of oxygen in normal body cells by a fermentation of sugar. All normal body cells meet their energy needs by respiration of oxygen, whereas [we have learned that] cancer cells meet their energy

---

[1]The Shpirt-Udalov team's experiments and findings were published by V/O MEDEXPORT, Moscow, in 1964. Under the aegis of the McNaughton Foundation, they were translated and published in pamphlet form in Los Angeles by Cancer Book House. An even larger volume of clinical evidence appears in a Soviet publication, *Vitamin B-15 (pangamic acid), Properties, Functions, and Use,* published in Moscow in 1965.

needs in great part by glucose fermentation. All normal body cells are obligate aerobes [i.e., they require oxygen to live] whereas all cancer cells are partial anaerobes [they thrive without oxygen].

"From the standpoint of the physics and chemistry of life," Warburg continued, "this difference between normal and cancerous cells is so great that one can scarcely picture a greater difference. Oxygen gas, the donor of energy in plants and animals, is dethroned in the cancer cell and is replaced by an energy-yielding reaction of the lowest living forms—namely, a fermentation of glucose."

According to Warburg's theory, then, cells face death when deprived of sufficient oxygen. To preserve themselves, some cells are able to switch metabolism and derive their energy from sugar fermentation. These cells become malignant. But if the cells were better able to withstand oxygen deprivation, they would have less need to switch to glucose fermentation for energy and would therefore be less likely to become malignant.

Therefore, in theory, if B-15 does indeed increase oxygen respiration, it should also be capable of preventing, if not curing, cancer by neutralizing the need of oxygen-starved cells to convert to glucose fermentation for energy. One can hardly imagine a more controversial or heatedly contested suggestion. Nor one requiring more expensive research to confirm or disprove. Some small, short-term, privately funded studies have been conducted on B-15's cancer-curing possiblities, but they produced no results. To establish the degree to which B-15 might *prevent* cancer with any certainty would require painstaking, long-term controlled studies, perhaps lasting twenty years or more; and, thus far, nobody has mounted such a major—and expensive—research program. On the contrary, the theory itself has been derided and declared unworthy of investigation.

After the first Soviet reports, the B-15 debate simmered along for several years in American medical and nutritional circles, with little change except that the Russians kept putting out more papers reporting new favorable findings. But it was not until the mid-1970's that Vitamin B-15 blossomed into something attracting widespread public attention in the United States. Then, in 1977, a book by a New York City doctor and nutritionist, *Dr. Atkins' Superenergy Diet,* catapulated B-15 into the popular arena where self-improvement, nutrition, and health had become the newest and hottest forms of chic. Dr. Robert Atkins, known as a "nutritionist to the stars," described B-15 as a health-enhancing, energy-producing, life-prolonging, disease-preventing agent. Suddenly B-15 was news.

As so often happens, the B-15 phenomenon blossomed first on the West Coast where B-15 suddenly became the hottest thing in California. Show business figures and physical-fitness bugs began to swear by its various benefits. It was Hollywood's sudden preoccupation with physiological health in 1977 that brought B-15 out of its earlier obscurity. It fitted right in with the whole complex of self-improvement, self-actualization, and self-realization movements that had developed in California in the form of Esalen, Arica, transcendental meditation, est, and the like. It was no longer okay just to strive for a healthy, vibrant soul; the body, being the temple of the spirit, deserved as much if not more attention. *Mens sana in corpore sano* became the credo of the new, new Hollywood.

Soon, stories about B-15's salubrious qualities spread to the Eastern show business and advertising worlds, and from there percolated down to the East Coast intelligentsia at large, although it remains a somewhat geographically localized phenomenon, concentrated in those cities with major communications and entertainment industries, with major outposts in the sports world. In Washington, D.C., for example, where the only industry is the government, querying a friend as to whether he has ever heard of B-15 is likely to elicit only a blank look and a vague question as to whether it's some new bomber aircraft.

Moreover, as too often happens, B-15 became an intensely polarized issue before *either* side had enough firm evidence to prove its case. Outside the Soviet Union, there has been little serious, systematic research focused specifically on B-15's possible benefits. Only now have some rigorously controlled scientific experiments been begun here in the United States, and although, as we shall see later in this book, their preliminary results are very encouraging indeed, their final findings won't be available for some time. Meanwhile, the battle lines in the B-15 debate have long since been laid down, more or less independently of the evidence.

The relative lack of hard scientific evidence has repeatedly put B-15's supporters at a disadvantage, leaving them without anything very firm to back up their beliefs and observations. Meanwhile, the FDA has based its own opposition to B-15 on this very lack of scientific evidence—yet no governmental agency has ever fielded the sort of research project that might conclusively disprove B-15's possibilities. The FDA maintains—correctly, in fact—that that is not its job and that it's up to the manufacturer to prove that his product is safe and effective. But at the same time the FDA has actively hindered anybody else's embarking upon such research, not scrupling in some cases to resort to what some call active harassment.

The result has been a debate that generates lots of heat but not much light, and that leaves the real facts about B-15 as unclear as ever. That sort of debate, however, is usually the hottest kind. Just listen to some of B-15's opponents:

"Pangamania!" quipped one doctor when queried about the life-saving and life-rejuvenating claims made for pangamic acid. "Like every other mania that has gripped this country regarding health, it too will pass when people discover there's nothing to it. B-15 is a load of malarkey!"

"As far as we're concerned," says FDA lawyer Ronald Craig, who was recently put in charge of enforcing laws against the substance's sale, "endorsing these pills would be like saying it's okay for the government to allow entrepreneurs to sell the public places in heaven because they insist that there's a life after death there. The evidence for the ability of B-15 to perform in the ways its pushers say it does is about as scientifically abundant as proof that there is a place called heaven where everybody goes after they die—or purgatory or hell.

"Look," Craig continues, "not one iota of objective scientific evidence has been produced to show that pangamic acid or pangamate is a genuine vitamin. Nor has anyone shown that it is a drug. All we've had is a bunch of claims with no supportive evidence, the Russians notwithstanding. You might observe that little has been heard from the Russians since that famous Shpirt report fifteen years ago. What's happened to all the additional research they promised? So all we have here is something that's extracted from a fruit pit that's neither a drug nor a vitamin, nor for that matter any kind of provable nutritional supplement. What is it, then? According to the statutes of our country, it is a food or food additive. Since it cannot be shown to provide any more of a nutritional benefit than the fruit from which it's extracted, namely the apricot, it cannot be considered a separate food. So, therefore, it can only be considered a food additive. And because it is a food additive, it must meet the safety standards for food additives which have been set by the government and which we are mandated by statute to guarantee and enforce. Forgetting the therapeutic and prevention and health-improving claims made for it, none of which have been medically substantiated, who knows what effects it has on the body when ingested, either occasionally or regularly? We have found that saccharin can have a deleterious effect on animals and have taken the appropriate measures to regulate its human use. We don't even know yet what if any effects pangamate might have. It might have none. It might have good ones. It might have bad ones which we wouldn't learn about until twenty years went by and people started dying of the progressively built-up effects. All we ask its advocates to show is that it won't have any short- or long-term toxic effects. When they can show that it won't, then we'll approve it for sale to the general public."

Nobody will question Ronald Craig's determination to uphold the laws and statutes of the United States. But it is worth analyzing his statement more closely, because it illustrates rather strikingly the way in which strategic omissions and prejudgments have distorted the B-15 debate. Let's begin with Craig's insistence that "not one iota of objective scientific evidence" has been presented in support of B-15's claims. Clearly, he dismisses the Soviet studies completely. Yet short of accusing the Soviets of outright, premeditated fraud—which, by the way, the FDA has indeed done in the past, going so far as to label the entire body of Soviet B-15 research a KGB plot to foment a miracle-drug hysteria in the United States—it is hard to maintain that there is absolutely *nothing* here worthy of notice. Moreover, as we shall see later in this book, there *is* hard, scientific evidence of B-15's beneficial powers beginning to come out of several serious, scientifically controlled studies now in progress in various places around the United States. (It is also worth noting that these studies have had to be conducted with something approaching classified security, for fear of FDA reprisals.) When these results are complete, it will be interesting to observe the hearing they get, given the remarkably entrenched hostility, *in the absence of any hard evidence one way or the other,* that has marked the reaction of medical and governmental circles in the past.

Then there's Craig's statement that the Soviets never did any further research on B-15 after the first reports back in the mid-1960's. Here it seems he is just flat-out wrong. "They don't read the literature!" exclaims Dr. Richard Passwater, a Virginia biochemist who has gotten extremely good results using B-15 in his work with professional athletes. "The Soviets put out a new paper on B-15 every six or eight weeks. All you have to do is keep abreast of the translations from the Russian in *Chemical Abstracts* and you'd see for yourself! And, good Lord, that's what the FDA is *supposed* to be doing! I don't know how they can justify that sort of statement at all."

Then there's the emphasis on B-15's possible toxicity. This has been the issue on which the FDA has officially based its opposition to B-15's sale and use. But if this were in fact the only obstacle in the way, it might have been removed long ago. It is interesting to note that another government agency concerned with public health seems quite convinced that B-15 won't hurt you. In the *Registry of Toxic Effects of Chemical Substances,* published by the U.S. Public Health Service of the Department of Health, Education, and Welfare, B-15 is listed as having an extremely low toxicity. The lethal dose for mice is cited as 255 mg/kg, administered intravenously, which means you'd practically have to replace the mouse's blood with B-15 before you could kill it. (Interestingly enough, this HEW publication lists B-15 as a "vitamin" despite the FDA's skepticism on that score.)

Moreover, there *is* laboratory evidence—from FDA contract work—that B-15 is about as close to completely nontoxic as any substance can come. Dr. Paul Buck, a biochemist and a member of the Vitamin and Mineral Board of the FDA, conducted lethal dosage tests of B-15 on animals at an FDA contract laboratory in Waverly, New York. According to Dr. Buck, the average person would have to ingest 21 pounds or more of B-15 tablets in a brief period of time to suffer toxic effects. By that time, the problem would not be the substance's toxicity but the digestive system's inability to handle that much *volume.* "Pangamic acid is completely safe to consume," asserts Buck, "and is neither the hoax nor the public ripoff the FDA has suggested." Why the FDA's attitude then? "Because of the overblown therapeutic claims being made for B-15 by some of its distributors." As far as Buck is concerned, pangamic acid *can* provide a nice energy boost and it may even be a disease preventive in certain respects, although he definitely does not consider it any sort of "miracle" vitamin or drug. "If it makes you feel good, go ahead and use it," he says. "It's not going to hurt you. Unless, of course, you put so much faith in it that you think it's the only thing you need and you don't have to take care of yourself. Other than that, we just don't know enough about what it does or how it does it. Some of the medical reports on it indicate"—Buck chooses his words carefully—"that it has some therapeutic properties, particularly when administered along with other therapeutically proven substances, in the treatment of certain diseases. But there is still not enough research to really say anything positive about it."

Well then, why doesn't the FDA accept Dr. Buck's report? Because, according to one version of the story, no FDA inspectors were invited to monitor those studies. "*I* know what they ran the safety studies on," says an ex-FDA inspector (who now is a strong advocate of B-15!), "and Dr. Buck knows what they ran the safety studies on, but the FDA doesn't—because Dr. Buck never submitted those safety studies until after they were done. Nobody had an opportunity to either establish what it was that was being done or to inspect it. They might not have done it anyway, but they never had the opportunity."

"Wrong!!" explodes Dom Orlandi at FoodScience/Da Vinci. "We had a meeting with the FDA, Paul Buck, and our chemist at the time. We told them, okay, we're going to run safety studies, and we told them that any time they wanted to come and see what these studies were doing, they were welcome. And they never showed up. Paul Buck even sent them a telegram putting all this in writing. And they never showed up."

It was, one recalls, Theodore Dreiser who remarked that truth was the first casualty of war . . .

What one is left with is a murky, emotional, heated debate in which the questions seem to outnumber the facts by a ratio of something like ten to one. For all the passion, controversy, and invective that B-15 has generated, most of the really important questions remain as yet unanswered. For that matter, a lot of energy seems to have been poured into keeping them from even being asked, either by hampering research or prejudging the issue. And one of the biggest unanswered questions is at the same time about the most basic: just what, in precise biochemical terms, *is* B-15? You might think we'd know, given all the fuss. But it turns out that there is a heated, unresolved debate on precisely that subject. It's tangled enough to warrant a chapter all to itself.

2

Will the Real B-15 Please Stand Up?

Okay, you figure, what the hell. It can't hurt me, and it *would* be nice not to feel so tired so often—so let's see what this stuff can do for me. So you go to your local health food store and ask for a bottle of "Vitamin B-15" and assume that whatever they sell you will be pretty much identical to what anybody else will get asking for the same thing somewhere else.

The only catch is, it might be something else entirely.

It's a matter of supply and demand. Early in 1978 *New York Magazine* published an article on Vitamin B-15 that attracted a lot of notice. Suddenly there was a huge demand for this hitherto obscure substance. Only there wasn't very much of it around because, until then, the market for it hadn't been all that big. Distributors found themselves unable to keep up with the demand, and as a result some twenty or more manufacturers jumped into this new and burgeoning market with products labeled "Vitamin B-15."

These products, however, differed considerably in chemical composition, and to ensure complete confusion, none of them specified on its label just what was in it, leaving the buyer very much in the position of purchasing a pig in a poke. And well might the buyer beware. Spectroscopic analyses done in 1978 at the State University of New York at Stonybrook showed that most of the B-15's on the market were composed primarily of one of two dissimilar substances: N,N-Dimethylglycine (or "DMG") or diisopropylamine (or "DIPA"), with some others consisting of an amino acid—glycine—and calcium gluconate. A few had jazzed up their formulae by adding niacinamide or—believe it or not—sugar.

Now, one of the hallmarks of the B-15 debate, as we shall see, is the fact that users of items labeled "B-15" have reported enormous variations in results, ranging all the way from nil to spectacular. To date, nobody has explained why this should be, and it has added fuel to the arguments of those who do not believe in B-15's possibilities that some people report that it does miraculous things for them while others report no effects at all. So far, nobody has tried to establish clearly which version of B-15 these people had been taking. Might this baffling irregularity of results have something to do with the fact that some people have been taking substances that simply were not Vitamin B-15 at all?

All of which lands us squarely in the middle of another battle in the War of B-15. This one rages *inside* the camp of B-15's own supporters, and the *casus belli* is the question: What, chemically speaking, is the "real" B-15? And if you have ever thought that scientists were a cool-headed, cold-blooded lot, you should try talking about this to some of the ones involved in the B-15 issue. Passions rise, charge leads to countercharge, and personal invective is not unknown. No abstract debate, this. It involves heartfelt opinions, professional reputations, and human emotions.

Exploring this matter can lead one into some fairly technical thickets of biochemistry. Sometimes it's hard for the layman to keep track of the arguments, because they come couched in complex biochemical explanations. The lay listener is bombarded with terms like "transmethylation," "intermediary metabolite," and "ester band." Yet these arguments, however abstruse they may seem to the uninitiated, lie at the core of the B-15 dispute, because they all bear on the central question: Assuming that *any* substance labeled "B-15" can do what its supporters say it can do, *which* substance is it, and just *how*, in biochemical terms, would it do what it does?

Dr. Ernest Krebs, Jr., insists that the only true B-15 is the substance he patented: glucono-dimethyl-amino-acetic acid. This formulation, however, is not commercially available. Why, one asks Dr. Krebs, should he neglect to make available something that he himself believes is of such enormous therapeutic value? Because, he says, its proper manufacture would require his constant personal attention since the method of synthesis is very slow, and he has not had the necessary time to devote to the task. Meanwhile, Dr. Krebs insists, his substance has not been duplicated by any other manufacturer, and therefore anything on the market right now calling itself "B-15" is a fraud.

But Dom Orlandi, whose firms FoodScience and Da Vinci Laboratories manufacture and sell their own formula of B-15 under the brand names Aangamik-15 and Gluconic-15, is equally insistent that the "real" B-15 is N,N-Dimethyl-glycine, which is the primary ingredient in this product. Orlandi, a shrewd, dark, stocky man with a pleasantly raucous sense of humor, is intensely dedicated to proving that DMG is of true health and nutritional value, and has poured his own considerable energies into that effort for many years now. He and his chief biochemist, Dr. Roger Kendall, a slender, intense young man who radiates enthusiasm for his work and for B-15, say that the reason Dr. Krebs has not marketed his version of B-15 is that his supposed method of synthesis is not just slow, it's impossible, and that Krebs is therefore in the embarrassing position of not being able to produce the very substance he claims to have discovered.

"I think Dr. Krebs *did* discover a natural substance in apricot pit kernels," says Kendall, "but I've had to conclude that the substance he synthesized differed from the substance he reported. Our attempts to synthesize his substance have produced an extremely unstable substance that could not be isolated in its pure form. Then, when we worked with the synthetic model, our results indicated that Krebs' reported procedure for isolating pangamic acid would instead have destroyed it!" Kendall and Orlandi are convinced that the "active ingredient," as it were, of B-15 is DMG, which, they say, is a naturally occurring substance in the cell, a known link in the chain of internal cell chemistry, and one that can dramatically improve the cell's nutritional environment and consequently the efficiency of all cellular reactions. Indeed, they say, what this whole search for the "real Vitamin B-15" leads one to is this natural metabolite, N,N-Dimethylglycine—which means that the whole idea of "Vitamin B-15" is a red herring that only muddies the issue, because there is no such thing.

"And let me tell you something," interrupts Dom Orlandi. "After that *New York Magazine* article came out, everybody and his dog put out something called 'B-15.' But right about that time my manufacturer tried to speed up our process by reversing a couple of critical steps, and the result was that I was rejecting batch after batch because of the presence of undesirable side products—if DMG isn't 99 percent pure, its efficacy is sharply reduced. My distributors were crying for supplies, because they could have sold everything I could have given them. But I wouldn't give them anything that had flunked our quality control tests. And ours is the only brand of 'B-15' on the market that consists of DMG. So during the height of the B-15 furor, there wasn't any *real* B-15 available to buy!"

How about DIPA, which seems to be the chief ingredient in most of the commercially available brands of B-15? Although its molecular structure is related to DMG, Dr. Kendall maintains that it behaves very differently in the cell. DMG's potency, he says, is directly related to its ability to act as a "methyl donor." (Here's where your basic cram course in biochemistry begins.) "Methyl" is a molecular fragment consisting of one carbon and three hydrogen atoms that can be transferred as a unit in a chemical reaction called "transmethylation." "Methyl donors" have these "methyl groups" attached to their molecule in such a way that they can be readily detached—in chemical parlance, they are "labile." Such labile methyl groups can do remarkable things in the body. For example, they can transform the hormone serotonin, which acts to constrict blood vessels, into a substance that does not constrict blood vessels—with considerable implications for the treatment of heart and circulatory ailments. Also, methyl groups convert the hormone norepinephrine into epinephrine (or adrenaline) and this is a heart stimulant. The end result would be an increase in blood flow, and that means more available oxygen.

The closer you look at it, in fact, the more important this process of transmethylation turns out to be. Methylation, we learn, is an indispensable chemical reaction in our metabolic processes. Vitamins, hormones, fats, proteins, and detoxification depend upon the transfer of the methyl group to complete their chemical cycle. Normal muscle chemistry cannot proceed without the functioning of methyl donors, because methylation is essential in protein metabolism to produce sarcosine and creatine—which is the substance that works to hold down lactic acid levels. The body cannot produce adrenaline without methylation. Choline is a methyl donor, and the lack of it can cause serious kidney dysfunction and fatty infiltration of the liver. Methylation is also extremely important in the body's ability to neutralize toxins. It is the vital process by which muscle energy continues to be liberated at the cellular level to form phosphocreatine—and without creatine or phosphocreatine muscle contraction, nerve conduction, and selective membrane permeability would not be possible.

Without methylation, in short, life would not exist. Unfortunately, the modern American diet is drastically lacking in foods that have labile methyl groups—for example, whole grains, cereal brans, and organ meats. And, thus far, no laboratory tests have been established to detect methylating deficiencies, so you may be methyl deficient and never know it, and never have any way of finding it out for sure. But if you are, *something* is likely to go wrong with you in time, because in the process of metabolism, the body constantly loses methyl groups by excreting them, and this means it has to keep getting new ones from methyl donors.

A lot of people now have come to believe that B-15 is the

most powerful natural methyl donor known. Dr. Kendall, however, insists that only one version of "B-15," namely, N,N-Dimethylglycine (DMG), can donate methyl groups in the necessary manner. "DIPA has more methyl groups than DMG does," he explains, "and therefore, on the face of it, one might expect that it would be an even better methyl donor than DMG. But those methyl groups are attached to the DIPA molecule in an entirely different manner from the way they are hooked on to the DMG molecule. They are not labile—which means that despite its greater number of methyl groups, DIPA cannot act as a methyl donor."

Kendall goes farther and maintains that DIPA might actually be a risky thing for some people to take. "DIPA is a vasodilator," he says. "That's something that expands and dilates blood vessels. It might cause a flush when you take it, the way niacin can do, and some people might even take that as evidence that something is really happening in their bodies. But for people with cardiovascular problems, that could be dangerous. In any event, DIPA is not going to do the things for you that DMG will, because of that inability to act as a methyl donor."

The confusion as to the chemical formulation of the "real" B-15 has added weight to the FDA's opposition to the substance in any form. As Dr. Allan Forbes, at one time acting associate director for nutrition and consumer sciences at the FDA, noted, "The flat truth of the matter is, to the best of our knowledge, you can't define the compound." Another FDA official in the Bureau of Foods said that B-15 "is not generally recognized as safe because it has no clear identity. . . . It's a mystery why it hasn't been described very carefully. The usual way to confirm an analysis is to synthesize it *de novo* and if you come up with the same substance, with the same biological activity, you can pretty much determine that what you thought it was *is* what it is." Still another FDA official, this one a chemist-nutritionist, points out that "there is considerable question as to how much pangamic acid is in these products, since no one is really monitoring them. People don't really know what they're getting. They don't know the chemical identity of it, nor how much is in the tablet they're actually purchasing. And there's nobody in the country checking on it. Nobody.''

The ex-FDA inspector quoted earlier—who now is convinced that B-15 (the DMG version) has helped both him and many other people to whom he has given bottles—nevertheless asserts very firmly that the FDA's position is absolutely proper—although the way they're pursuing it might not be. ''The Kefauver Amendment, which was passed in 1964, says you can't manufacture a product for interstate commerce without establishing its safety and efficacy,'' he begins. ''Now if you read a B-15 label, the first thing you see is that it contains calcium pangamate. But there's no official definition of 'calcium pangamate' in the United States, and no manufacturer who claims his product is calcium pangamate has bothered to establish one. So nobody officially knows what they're dealing with.

''Furthermore,'' he goes on, ''I don't know if anybody could economically *afford* to legalize B-15. For example, if one of the manufacturers finally got tired of all this and said, okay, we're going to spend half a million dollars getting an approved new drug application, then once he'd done that, three thousand other guys could say 'me, too' on his dough and compete actively in his marketplace. So from the economic standpoint he's better off if the stuff is never legalized!''

For that very reason, says Dom Orlandi, FoodScience/Da Vinci has hitherto been reluctant to come out and say that their product is in fact N,N-Dimethylglycine—because that's a natural substance, and you can't patent natural substances. ''Once we went public with the fact,'' he notes, ''then everybody could swipe our formula, although they'd have their work cut out for them to get the manufacturing process right —we're the only ones who know how to make the stuff in proper potency and purity. So why are we coming out now and saying our product is DMG? Because since that *New York*

Magazine article, the market's being flooded by a whole lot of cheap, ineffective brands—all of which are mostly DIPA—and they'll end by giving a bad name to *everything* called B-15. I mean, how would you feel if you bought this bottle of so-called B-15, and spent good money for it, and it didn't do a thing for you? So we made the decision to reveal our formula, because if we didn't, it'd hurt us worse in the long run."

Have doctors using B-15 with their patients noticed any differences in the effectiveness of various versions of the substance? "Absolutely!" exclaims Dr. Robert Atkins, the New York nutritionist who helped put B-15 on the map. "There's a lot of stuff around that is not B-15 at all. In fact, for a while after that *New York Magazine* article came out, I quit giving it to my patients because it had gotten so popular that I couldn't count on consistent quality. I treat a lot of people complaining of fatigue, and I find that B-15 is very good at regulating their blood sugar. I've found that the best formulation is the calcium salt of N,N-Dimethylglycine." Dr. Bernard Rimland, head of the Institute for Child Behavioral Research in San Diego, also uses this version in his work with autistic children.

On the other hand, Dr. Richard Passwater, the previously mentioned Virginia biochemist whose extensive work with professional athletes convinced him that B-15 is of enormous value in building stamina and oxygen capability, uses both DIPA and DMG in his work. "Each seems to have different effects," he says. "DIPA probably uses a different route, and it seems to have a stimulating cardiovascular effect. DMG probably is easier for the body to handle. Heart patients respond well to both. On the other hand, athletes seem to do better on DMG."

Why care about all this in the first place? Why the preoccupation with what—if anything—happens inside the cell when either DIPA, or DMG, or anything else for that matter, is introduced into the body system? The answer is that the cell and its ability to perform its tasks efficiently are the foundation of body function and health. We are all taught as youngsters to perceive the human body as a collection of bones, connective tissues, and organs encased in an envelope of skin. But to understand the body better, as well as the manner in which it functions, we need to refine that perception. A more fruitful way of viewing the body is in its most fundamental form: as a structure composed of trillions of cells encased in a skin envelope that is itself made up of countless cells.

The cell and its nucleus is the basic form of human life. We all start our embryonic existence as single cells that rapidly multiply themselves in the womb to form the substance and shape of our human organism. The gradual transformation from embryo to fetus during gestation, and then from fetus to infant ready to enter the world, is nothing more than a process of cell division and multiplication. By the time we are born, our biology—which is to say, our cellular mechanics—is the engine of our existence.

But there is more to us than just biology. There is also chemistry, which is the mode by which our biological engines are fueled and made to live and function. Chemistry is a function of the glands and organs of the body, all of which are composed of cells. When we are in the womb, our cells are initially fed, fueled, and proliferated through our mother's chemistry. Once we are born, however, our own chemistries take over to continue our cellular growth and functioning.

The primary component of our chemistry is metabolism. Metabolism is the dual process by which nutrients from outside the body (principally food, water, and air) are converted into waste and expelled. The basic functions of metabolism are to provide energy to the cells, to keep them in a state of healthy natural suspension, and to repair them when they break down. The fundamental mechanisms of metabolism are the cardiopulmonary system, the digestive system, the bloodstream, and the various organs and glands of nutrient manufacture and waste excretion. And the primary medium of the metabolic process is the circulatory system, itself a vast cellular network, which carries nutrients and oxygen to every cell in the body and which transfers waste materials to the organs of excretion.

Every individual cell in the body is a complex, dynamic

chemical factory. Each cell takes chemicals into itself, changes its size or shape according to production requirments, and creates other chemicals that it transfers to other cells. What's even more remarkable, it performs all these reactions, many of which would take very high temperatures to complete in a laboratory, at the strikingly low temperature of 98.6°F. Of course, of the many kinds of cells—muscle cells, brain cells, heart cells, blood cells, and so on—each has its own job to do. A bone cell does not take in the same chemicals as a blood cell; it does not look like a blood cell; and it does not manufacture the same chemicals. But the fact remains that every cell is an elaborate microscopic chemical factory. And though various cells perform various vital biochemical functions, each cell requires oxygen to carry out its performance. This is what every cell has in common: it needs oxygen to live and perform. Oxygen is what gives it the energy to carry out its biochemical tasks.

Oxygen is carried to the cells through the blood after being processed through the cardiopulmonary system (the lungs and heart). The essential chemical nutrients of the cells—vitamins, minerals, amino acids, carbohydrates, fats, and others—are also transported through the blood after being extracted from the foods we ingest. The blood-supply system, then, is a key element in the health of the body's cells.

The blood-supply system is itself constituted of cells. During the natural aging process, the cells of the lungs deteriorate and lose their ability to process oxygen into the bloodstream. When less oxygen flows through the blood and reaches the cells of the other vital organs of the body, deterioration in these cells begins. These organs, deprived of their required cell energy, in turn suffer a progressive diminution in their power to perform their biochemical metabolic functions.

In our modern industrialized world, lung-cell deterioration begins much earlier than it otherwise would in the natural aging process. Hence, premature general body-cell deterioration results as oxygen supply is reduced. The reduction in oxygen supply diminishes the ability of vital organs to function at peak capacity, causing the cells of these organs to seek their energy from other sources—that is, to change their basic metabolism. Once they do this, they become ''alien'' cells and tend by their own chemical processes to transform surrounding cells into cells like themselves. With the cellular balance upset, degeneration and disease follow. The entire process is also helped along by certain staples in our standard modern diet that tend to constrict and harden the linings of our blood-supply vessels and organs, further reducing oxygen supply.

This is, of course, a simplified account, but according to a consensus of medical experts, this general process is how degenerative disease develops. It is also the process that medical proponents of Vitamin B-15 believe the substance can reverse.

Still, the question remains: *How* would it do that? We need to know how B-15—whichever version one chooses to regard as authentic—acts in the cell, because only that sort of hard, scientific information will allow us to know what B-15's ''true'' formula is and what we may or may not expect it to do for us. And, so far, we are still in the realm of theory, and hotly contested theory at that.

One theory proposes that B-15 stimulates the suprarenal hypophysis—a tiny gland that seems to play a role in removing many oxygen-consuming waste products from the bloodstream. This causes wastes to be eliminated from the body more quickly. As a result, less oxygen is consumed by the wastes and more oxygen remains for cellular metabolism. Since it is from this accumulation of waste that oxygen-starved cells get their substitute energy, thus transforming themselves into alien cells, retarding waste accumulation would cause oxygen insufficiency (hypoxia) to do less damage, and would leave a longer period of time for normal oxygen metabolism to be reestablished without damage to the organ.

Another theory suggests that B-15 promotes increased oxygen capacity in the blood itself by stimulating respiratory enzymes in the metabolic system. Thus, it would not only retard cell-waste accumulation during reduced oxygen nourishment, it also would provide increased oxygen to every cell in the body, further normalizing them and preventing them from having to seek other, disease-inducing sources of energy.

A third theory says that B-15 donates methyl groups to potentially toxic substances, thereby rendering them harmless. Thus, less oxygen is consumed in detoxification metabolism and more oxygen remains available for cellular metabolism. "I'd love to see some radioactive studies done on the basis of this hypothesis," says Dr. Richard Passwater. "By tagging the molecules, you could see if B-15 enters the body chemistry from methyl groups or on behalf of the whole molecule. It would tell us a lot about what B-15 does and how."

Dr. Roger Kendall at FoodScience/Da Vinci says they're planning to do just that. "The full implications of di-methylglycine are not yet known," he remarks. "It would be nice if I could give you a complete blow-by-blow description of everything that happens in the metabolic cycle when DMG is introduced, but the search just hasn't come that far yet. But we do have a very good idea of what's happening in terms of methyl groups, and sometime in the near future we plan to actually do some tagging experiments with DMG where we tag the methyl groups with radioactive carbon and then follow it through the body by tracking the natural radioactivity associated wtih Carbon 14."

Although Ernest Krebs insists vehemently that only his formula can produce B-15's claimed benefits, he offers little exact explanation as to how it might behave inside the cell, aside from asserting that it "increases oxygen uptake." Since this does not answer the basic question of *how* it does that, however, it leaves the listener as much in the dark as ever.

Dr. Kendall offers the explanation that DMG, Da Vinci Laboratories' candidate for the "real" B-15, functions as an "active intermediary metabolite," which energizes and improves energy production within the cell. He explains it this way: "When you have a cellular substance, a nutrient of some sort, most are changed from one to another in the cell. This is done by 'metabolites.' An 'intermediary' metabolite is one that has a source within the cell; that is, it is formed *in* the cell by other precursors and is converted to other substances in the cell. Conceivably, if you know the exact structures of these key metabolites, you could introduce substances somewhere along the chain of reactions and alter the whole chain. We believe that DMG is such a metabolite, altering the rate and direction of various chemical transformations within the cell.

"Some things like Vitamin C, for instance, function intact in the cell," Dr. Kendall notes. "But DMG seems to do what it does by *falling apart*—that is, by giving up its methyl groups." Then he begins to get technical again. "DMG will enhance the production of ATP, or adenosine triphosphate," he explains. "That's the major energy supplier for most of the biochemical energy processes in the cell. Furthermore, we know through animal studies that by this process of methyl transfer DMG will enhance the synthesis of creatine and phosphocreatine—which in turn helps hold down lactic acid build-up, the cause of muscle fatigue. Transmethylation, moreover, is significant in the biochemical synthesis of several key nutritional substances, including adrenaline, phosphocreatine, methionine, and choline. In fact, a *secondary* effect of adding DMG to your diet may be that you save your choline. That's because the choline would no longer be needed for making DMG, as it now is in the choline cycle in the cell, and so it would be available for other things—like, for example, preventing fatty infiltration of the liver."

This, too, of course, is still only a theory, and as such is hotly contested by others, notably Dr. Krebs, who dismisses this entire line of reasoning as specious, because he considers DMG a worthless imitation of the "true" B-15 he maintains he discovered. But the fact remains that nobody has yet done the necessary research to test these various theories and discover which, if any, of them is correct. As we shall see later in the book, some experiments are now at last in progress.

All of these theories at least have one thing in common: they all center on the relationship between B-15 and oxygen. B-15's supporters contend that daily dosages of pangamic acid can help counter the deteriorating effects on the body's cells of modern diet and environment by correcting the internal oxygen imbalances caused by these factors. Because B-15 produces more oxygen in the blood system, the theory goes, cells receive more respiration and energy than normal, which enables them to perform their chemical functions at optimum levels. Being able to perform at these levels—the levels nature demands for good health—the cells have no need to seek other forms of energy and thus no need to become alien and disease-prone.

In addition to all this educated guessing there are, of course, the Soviet studies, which have been going on for several years now and which continue to report very favorable results, though many members of the American scientific and medical community find them unconvincing. Apart from the somewhat emotional reaction of dismissing the Russian results as suspect solely on the grounds of their source, other more considered objections to them have arisen on two accounts: first, the Soviets' vagueness as to the precise chemical composition of the pangamic acid used in their experiments; and, second, certain flaws in their basic experimental design.

It seems that one can't quite tell from the Soviet reports just what it was that they used under the name of "calcium pangamate" in their studies. Dr. Krebs says that it was the potassium salt of pangamic acid. But Dr. Kendall says that attempts to discover from the Soviet accounts the exact chemical composition of their substance have failed and that Food-Science/Da Vinci Laboratories' efforts to synthesize the Soviet compound have yielded very low purities, far below what would be necessary to identify the substance scientifically. "The Soviets have always been somewhat elusive on the subject of the chemistry of their pangamic acid," he remarks. "Interestingly enough, in the late 1960's, Dr. I. N. Garkina seemed to intimate in a paper she gave at a symposium in the U.S.S.R. that DMG is the active ingredient in B-15, when she stated that it was the intermediary metabolite that forms on the breakdown of the pangamic structure. But aside from that one mention, the Soviets have carefully avoided coming out in the open with the structure of their substance. I'm only guessing, of course, but it's my opinion that the reason they avoid the matter is that they want to protect that patent they filed here in 1975 on their version of pangamic acid—and since DMG is a natural substance, it's not patentable.'' (There just might be something in that, inasmuch as it would be far from the first time the Soviets had shown themselves to be canny players of the capitalist business game.)

Another reason for the suspicion with which many in the United States treat the Soviet studies is that, in such matters, the American biomedical community ordinarily considers the only fully reliable form of experimental design to be the ''double blind,'' a technique not in common use in Russia. In a double-blind experiment, the experimental subjects are divided into two groups. One group, the ''test group,'' is given the substance to be tested; the other, the ''control group,'' is given a placebo, which is identical to the pill the test group is receiving in all respects except for its active ingredient. Neither the test group, the control group, nor the people administering the pills and collating the data knows who has been getting what. In this way, the so-called placebo effect, whereby some people will get better just because they *think* they are taking something to help them, is screened out. This, however, is not a procedure the Soviets rely on extensively and, by and large, they have not used control groups of any sort in their B-15 studies. Consequently, many in the United States find the Soviet results to be suspect simply on the basis of their research design.

Outside of the Soviet work, there has been only a handful of controlled medical studies of B-15's effects, so we are working with pretty limited data all around. But even if we had finally established firmly that B-15 was indeed of nutritional and therapeutic utility, we would still find ourselves facing some other questions just as important—namely, does B-15 do what it does in and of itself? or does it depend upon its interaction with other nutritional supplements? If so, which ones and in what amounts? This could be called the ''synergism question,'' and we don't have any precise answers to it either.

Again, there is some scattered evidence on the subject.

Doctors who use B-15 with their patients generally agree that it works best in conjunction with a full nutritional regimen. Several mention its utility in conjunction with chelation therapy, a form of therapy that is gaining growing attention in the treatment of arteriosclerosis. It is a technique whereby a synthetic amino acid called ethylenediamine tetra-acetic acid (EDTA) is given intravenously in the patient's arm over an interval of approximately four hours, and repeated as needed. EDTA has the property of binding with the calcium in the patient's bloodstream. The blood then reacts to maintain its calcium level; in order to do so, it draws on the calcium contained in the plaque that builds up on the blood vessel walls of arteriosclerosis victims. This breaks the plaque up and allows it to be dislodged. Apparently, the beneficial effect of chelation therapy in allowing increased blood flow through previously obstructed blood vessels combines well with B-15's apparent ability to increase the amount of oxygen available for that blood to carry to the tissues.

Vitamins A and E may also enhance B-15's effects. The Soviets reported that they used something called "Aevit" along with B-15 in their work, but—in another of their tantalizing omissions—neglected to explain just what, precisely, Aevit was. To make matters more confused, their research design did not attempt to determine the degree to which the benefits they ascribed to B-15 were dependent upon the interaction among all these substances, or, as some have charged, due to the Aevit, whatever it was, and not to the B-15 at all.

When one begins talking to doctors and medical practitioners in the United States, one finds the same problem repeated. Time and again, the people one interviews report good results from using B-15; but, nearly always, they have been using it in conjunction with other nutritional substances and therapeutic techniques. On occasion, one will be told of a patient who had been on a fully established regimen *before* B-15 was added, and the doctor is then able to say that the good results began after B-15 was introduced. But this tends to be the exception.

Dom Orlandi is quick to assert that his brand of B-15 works best in conjunction with a comprehensive program of vitamin and mineral supplements. He recommends that it be taken in conjunction with his multivitamin supplement, Omni (which consists of a really stupefying array of vitamins and minerals in blitz quantities), and another product called Perna, which is very rich in seaborne minerals. "A lot of professional sports teams"—here he reels off a long list of major-league teams in both the United States and Canada—"buy our Omni and Perna as well as our Aangamik-15. Moreover, they buy them in quantity. I'm assuming that the reason they are spending the money to do that is because they are getting results."

Well, as things stand now, you pays your money and you takes your choice. The more you get into the B-15 debate, the more questions and the fewer answers you find. Still, it seems pretty certain that *something* out there is the "real" B-15—whatever that may be—because a lot of people have reported some really remarkable results from taking this puzzling substance. Let's hear some of their stories.

3

Sports, Stamina, and Staying Power

The primary physical requisite of most competitive athletic endeavors is muscle stamina. Boxing fans are accustomed to seeing fighters grow arm-weary after four or five rounds of furious swinging. Joggers know all too well the frustration of exhausted, crampy leg muscles when the mental will to continue running remains. Weightlifters and bodybuilders are intimately acquainted with the manner in which a given muscle absolutely refuses to continue to function after a certain number of repetitions. And any athlete who is a regular smoker is keenly aware of how quickly his muscles will become fatigued when engaging in a strenuous sport. Why? It all has to do with oxygen.

The muscles of our body are, like everything else, composed of cells. And like everything else, they demand oxygen from the lungs and circulatory system to function. As continued or repeated stress is placed on a muscle, it demands more and more oxygen to maintain its level of function. The cardiopulmonary system tries to furnish the increased supply of oxygen, but for any number of reasons may not be able to. Lung cells may have deteriorated as a result of smoking or other environmental causes so that an insufficient amount of oxygen is processed into the heart. Or the heart may not be capable of pumping sufficient amounts of oxygen into the arteries to satisfy the working muscle's demands. Or the arteries may be narrowed by deposits of fatty plaques that reduce or constrict the flow of oxygen to the capillaries that feed oxygen to the muscle. In many cases, all these phenomena and more interact to starve the straining muscle of its oxygen-nourishment demands.

What occurs then is what is known in athletic circles as "oxygen debt." As a muscle is being used, it expends energy. In other words, every time a muscle contracts, its fibers, which are networks of microscopic cells, require energy to sustain the contraction, and they are constantly using up energy. The necessary energy is provided by the fresh oxygen and chemical nutrients fed into the muscle by the blood vessels. As the oxygen is used in the muscle's cells, the cells manufacture a waste chemical that is meant to be expelled through the return flow of blood. This by-product is called lactic acid. Under normal conditions, the lactic acid is carried off as waste at the same rate that fresh oxygen is being supplied, so that the two substances exist in a kind of natural balance in the muscle's cells. But when the muscle is placed under stress and insufficient oxygen is supplied to meet the energy demands of that stress, the lactic acid begins to accumulate in the cells. Deprived of sufficient oxygen for its energy, the muscle then seeks to metabolize the lactic acid. As a result, the cells of the muscle temporarily begin to "alienize" themselves. The consequence is at first fatigue, and then, if stressed long enough, spasms and cramps. The muscle is in oxygen debt and can no longer function in a natural way. The owner of the muscle has to stop what he is doing and rest, allowing oxygen to build up again to dissipate the lactic acid, before he can resume the activity.

Aside from polishing their skills, the reason competitive athletes must train is basically to increase their muscle stamina. Many otherwise ordinary athletes have become extraordinary because they have been able to expand their muscle stamina—indeed, their entire body stamina—beyond that of naturally more gifted athletes. Such stamina expansion consists of nothing more than enhancing and improving the oxy-gen-supply system to the muscles. In recent times, B-15 has become an important, and, many believe, a successful adjunct to such training.

It all began in the Soviet Union. After the Shpirt report was released, detailing the oxygen-increasing qualities of pan-gamic acid, Soviet Olympic coaches consulted with physicians involved in the B-15 medical studies and came away with the recommendation that they experiment with B-15, or calcium pangamate, as a daily supplement in the diets of the athletes they were preparing for the 1968 Olympics. The reason B-15 must be taken regularly—daily or two to three times a day—is that it is a water-soluble substance like the B-Complex vita-mins and Vitamin C. Fat-soluble vitamins such as A and E store themselves in the body, but water-soluble ones do not, surpluses being shed by the various organs and glands of excretion. Such substances must be steadily renewed to have the continuing desired effects.

The Soviets shared their hopes for B-15 with other Com-munist countries, notably East Germany, training to compete in the 1968 Olympics. Although the Russians did better than ever before in the games, the East Germans, who had hitherto been poor contenders in the Olympics and who were even more avid than the Soviets in their inclusion of an intensive B-15 intake regimen in their training programs, suddenly star-tled the world with their feats, particularly in the endurance competitions. Especially outstanding were East Germany's women athletes, whom many accused of training on male hormones. The Communist coaches reacted to such accusa-tions with reticent smiles, not wanting to share their secret with the West.

It was not long, however, before the secret leaked. Soon, scores of medical-nutritional practitioners in North America and Western Europe were making note of the Communists' reliance on B-15 for athletic purposes. In the meantime, Rus-sian researchers began to conduct organized, controlled studies on swimmers and rowers. Their findings showed a definite decrease in the build-up of lactic acid in the muscles of the athletes who had been placed on B-15 regimens.

The issue even got tangled up with the question of American military preparedness. In 1969 the Russians began to add B-15 to the diets of selected Red Army combat regiments in an experiment designed to determine whether or not the substance was capable of inducing better fighting performance on the part of the Soviet soldier. When this became known, the U.S. Army joined with the CIA in an effort to learn if B-15 improved performance and courage in such combat sports as boxing and wrestling—the assumption being that if it did, then front-line Soviet soldiers who had been consuming B-15 for several years would experience similar improvement in performance in combat situations, thereby gaining an edge over NATO fighting troops in Europe. Knowing that the Communist-bloc nations intended to train their athletes on B-15 for the 1972 Olympics, the Army and the CIA sent a team of special secret observers to the games to monitor Communist-bloc boxers and wrestlers in action and decide if their performances signaled marked increases in courage, determination, and staying power over those demonstrated in previous Olympiads. If they did, the Americans in charge of the project planned to recommend that B-15 be incorporated, much like the legendary saltpeter of previous army generations, in the foods dispensed at mess halls throughout the military base system.

What the Army was really worried about was the fact that its enlisted ranks were becoming increasingly populated by young men from the lower and deprived economic classes. Those in charge of training and deploying these tens of thousands of young men had begun to entertain serious reservations about their motivation and determination to fight at full tilt for their country should they ever be thrust into combat situations against Soviet and other communist troops. The Army wanted to learn whether the Russian, East German, and other boxers representing the Communist bloc were able to best the American team through the reinforced courage and energy supposedly provided by several years of B-15 consumption. If the communist fighters prevailed over the Americans, the hypothesis ran, the U.S. Army faced a crisis.

As it happened, the American team acquitted itself admirably and the Army-CIA mission to Munich returned without any recommendations about incorporating B-15 into the diet of the American soldier. Nevertheless, because the Soviets were still using it, certain selected American infantry battalions were fed B-15 in their food, without their knowledge, in an experiment conducted at various army posts in the United States and Europe during 1973 and 1974. As these dietary experiments progressed, Army scientists were dispatched to the field to measure the results during war games and maneuvers. Although the results were never wholly documented, certain data pointed to the conclusion that those infantry battalions that had been fed diets supplemented by B-15 generally performed better than those that had not.

Meanwhile, back in the sports world, word of B-15 was spreading. Ironically, the first observable results of using B-15 with athletes in North America came not from humans but from horses—thoroughbred race horses. A wealthy Canadian race-horse owner heard about the Soviet studies, and, on a hunch, instructed his trainer to begin feeding B-15 to several of the less distinguished performers in his stable. The results were startling. Two of the horses became consistent winners within months, and two more performed far above their previous form. Within the year, as the information spread, trainers all over Canada were dosing their horses' oats with pulverized calcium pangamate.

Dr. Richard Passwater was among the first Americans to look into the phenomenon. He claims that his experiments showed that the oxygen-increasing properties of B-15 not only retarded lactic acid build-up in the muscles of athletes, but that they also served to retain muscle glycogen, or reserve fuel, thus markedly enhancing the athlete's endurance and stamina. He brought his data to George Allen, the newly appointed coach of the Washington Redskins football team who had recruited a squad of experienced but aging players. Allen, celebrated in professional football circles as a man who would do anything to gain an edge, approved Passwater's suggestion that B-15 be included in the team's regular training regimen. When the Redskins surprised the country by performing well beyond anyone's expectations year after year during the mid-1970's, some insiders gave Passwater the credit.

As word spread, professional athletes all over the country began using B-15 in the mid-1970's. At the time it was regarded simply as a "pep" pill and was considered by its users as something illegal and therefore risky to talk about. Since then, however, things have loosened up, although the teams themselves are still somewhat reticent about admitting openly that they use B-15 in their training regimens, because of the possibility that the FDA might then end up designating B-15 a drug—which would make it illegal to use in professional sports. But individual players are often more outspoken, and one can now find dozens of athletes who either use B-15 regularly now or once did so to improve their stamina and endurance. Most are competitors in the more strenuous and energy-draining sports such as basketball, football, lacrosse, soccer, tennis, and track. Their experiences are extremely intriguing because of the extraordinarily wide range of results they report. Some swear by it. Others find it disappointing.

Major-league ball teams—both football and baseball—may not be quite ready to swear by B-15 in public, but they have gotten interested enough to incorporate it increasingly into their training programs. "The teams are starting to get into nutrition now instead of just the old steak-and-potatoes routine," says a young FoodScience salesman who has begun getting very good orders from big-league teams in both the United States and Canada. "One leading East Coast team" (he mentions the name but insists on confidentiality due to the team's worries about possible troubles with government agencies) "has been using Gluconic-15 since just before the play-offs and throughout the last part of the season. They really like the results. The trainer tells me that most of the players report having an increased energy supply, longer endurance, more stamina when needed, and better recovery after big games. A Canadian team tells me that all their players are definitely feeling a lot better on B-15. They have greater endurance, and do a lot better in the second half of the game, especially their running backs. They've reordered four or five times now over a period of about three months.

"One major NFL team is so interested in it that they are planning to set up a serious research program with us," he goes on. "They'll start by running blood tests, lactic acid level studies, and hair analyses with all their players. Then they'll work into a nutritional program including Gluconic-15 and other nutritional items and monitor the results. The ultimate aim is to design an individualized nutritional program for each player using B-15."

Individual professional athletes frequently report spectacular results from taking B-15. Françoise Durr, for example, swears by it. A highly ranked professional tennis player, this Frenchwoman claims that regular B-15 usage has been a boon to her career. Although not as technically skilled in the fundamentals of the game as some of her higher ranked peers, she is noted for her ability to wear opponents down by pure endurance and credits her success to the greater staying power she possesses as a result of B-15 intake.

A survey of athletes in other sports turned up similar findings. Several competitors in the 1977 New York Daily News Golden Gloves amateur prizefights were found to have trained on B-15, among other nutrients and food additives. Several attributed their success to calcium pangamate, remarking on such benefits as increased punching power and reductions in that bane of all boxers—arm-weariness. One even said that he was convinced he had become better able to take punches, that a punch that might earlier have knocked him out now only dazed him.

Interviews with the weightlifters and bodybuilders at a New York health club turned up similar testimonials to B-15. "Since I started on it," said one pretender to the Mr. Universe crown, "my development has speeded up tremendously. With more oxygen getting to my muscles, I can go longer at any exercise. The difference is amazing, and it all happened in a period of two to three weeks after I started taking four 200-mg hits of B-15 a day." He demonstrated, lifting a 110-pound dumbbell and beginning a biceps-building routine. "Used to be I could lift this thing ten, eleven times before my arm would quit. Now watch." He completed 25 repetitions without strain. "I could go on for another ten or eleven before it begins to hurt," he said. "Instead, I'll move it up to 140 pounds." He accomplished ten repetitions at 140 pounds, straining somewhat on the last two. "Without B-15," he concluded, "I'd still be a year away from being able to do that."

Two of the most grueling sports in the world are long-distance running and swimming. "You've heard of the loneliness of the long-distance runner," one marathon racer said to me. "Well, since I've been taking B-15, I'm no longer lonely. When I run, I feel I've got this little friend inside me running with me. That's what it's done for me. I noticed the difference almost immediately. My times started getting better and, at the same time, the effort became less. A year ago, I couldn't finish a [26-mile] marathon in under four hours because I'd always come to a point in a race where I'd just have to slow down to a walk for about two miles until I got some gas back. But now I'm under three hours and I never have to slow down. The more B-15 I pump into myself, the better my times are becoming. And there's never that tremendous letdown for the next few days that I used to experience. I used to have to practically stay in bed for two or three days after a race or else I'd pass out from dizziness. Absolute oxygen depletion. And I couldn't move my bowels or urinate, so you can imagine all the poisons that built up in me. I'd be literally sick for a week after. But now, with B-15, I'm as good as new the day after a race, and I can go out and do a 10-mile training run without a qualm."

Quintana Secors is the pseudonym of a celebrated long-distance swimmer who prefers not to be publicly associated with B-15 because she recently signed a contract to endorse a well-known conventional food product to which she will be crediting much of her athletic stamina. Yet she privately swears by B-15 as the reason for her recent endurance successes in the water. "In addition to all the normal things you'd expect it to do for you," she says, "it has solved the biggest problem any endurance swimmer has. And that's this business of hallucinations. With me it has always been there, no matter how many conventional nutrients I took during a swim. I'd just get to a point where nothing would stem the oxygen starvation. It was as if all the oxygen I had left in my body was going into my arms and being stolen from every other part of me. My legs would go numb, my back would seize up, but, worst of all, my brain would fly out of my head. I'd enter a dream world of hallucination, and the images would become so distracting in their horror and scariness that I'd want to quit the swim. I'd go into panic, begin swallowing sea water as if I was bent on destroying myself, in order to avoid going on. But now that's all a thing of the past. Sure, I still get the occasional hallucination, but it's never bad and I'm always on top of it. There's always a part of my brain that remains in control, so that I'm aware of what's going on at all times."

A 56-year-old New York man reports similar help from B-15 in his swimming. (He uses the DMG version of B-15.) "I swim Masters Competition competitively," he says. "I tried for maybe two years to swim a half-mile in under fifteen minutes. No go. Then I took this stuff for three days, and on the fourth day I went down to a YMCA with my wife and a whole bunch of other guys, and I put three halves back to back, and *all* of them were under fifteen minutes! I think that's pretty good, especially when you figure that people my age don't improve—whatever stamina you've got at 56 is probably what you're stuck with.

"You're not talking about a lot of time—maybe eight, ten, twelve seconds—but in a swimming pool that's half a length. I wasn't swimming any faster. I just wasn't loitering around gasping for breath on the turns.

"I've given a lot of this stuff away to friends," he goes on breezily. "I'd say it's about 80 percent effective. I know it's effective with me. I've got one guy, for example, who's the director of counseling down at a college on Long Island. He's got a couple of doctorates in psychology. He's a broken-down over-age jock, runs eight, nine miles a day, and he will swear to you that B-15 has changed his life. What he says is that he now has the energy to conduct a private practice—you know, he does marital counseling, and frolics with some freaks in an office in his home. But he says he now has the energy to do what he does at school, run, *and* conduct a private practice, and he never did that before."

B-15 seems to do good things for race horses too. Bruce Muir, another young FoodScience/Da Vinci salesman, reports that a veterinarian in the Midwest, who has seven race horses of his own, started feeding them FoodScience's supplement for horses, Spur 15. Then he tracked the horses' performances carefully for a full year, taking blood tests periodically along the way. "Before he started giving the horses our supplement," Muir relates, "one of the horses customarily won his races while the rest were used to coming in at best second or third. After he put them all on the supplement, several of the horses that usually came in second or third were starting to win, while the ones that had usually never even placed were starting to place. The blood tests showed that there was a rise in the hemoglobin count in their blood.

"It wasn't that the horses were running faster," notes Muir. "It was just that they were now able to run as fast as they were capable of running for longer periods of time. That's because the DMG kept the circulation going in their legs. When a horse gets tired, it's not usually because of winding. It's because there's lactic acid build-up in the legs that's tiring the horse. The reason that lactic acid builds up is that the 'frog' is not functioning properly. The 'frog' is the soft pad in the middle of the horse's hoof, and in the natural state its function is to act sort of like a bellows and pump the blood back up into the horse's leg each time he pushes off the ground. When you shoe a horse, you protect his hoof, but you also prevent the frog from doing its intended job. So the circulation in his legs will suffer. DMG works to counteract that problem."

Judy Juhring is a wealthy young widow and avid horsewoman who maintains a large farm in North Carolina where she breeds horses for fox hunting and steeplechase racing. She first came across B-15 when she learned that her farm manager was treating injured horses with it. "According to him," she says, "it was very effective in promoting the healing of muscle, ligament, and tendon injuries. When a horse pulls a tendon in his leg, the conventional treatment is to 'fire' it—that is, insert hot needles into the area to create a counter-irritant that will in turn bring more blood to the area and hasten healing. Well, my manager had run into some Russian trainers who were visiting the United States touring horse farms; they told him about B-15 as an alternative to this method. He tried it on a couple of my hunting horses and found that it worked. The horses recuperated much more quickly on B-15 than when they were fired. I was told that it had something to do with the B-15 getting more oxygen-saturated blood into the injured tissues. Anyway, the difference in healing time was remarkable. Word got around and pretty soon people all over the fox-hunting world were using the stuff on their horses. Then we began to hear of horses that had been treated with B-15 suddenly becoming much better jumpers than they had been before. The B-15, some said, not only increased oxygen to damaged tissues, thereby speeding up healing, but increased oxygen to all the other muscles. The horses were becoming more powerful and could go for longer and longer distances without tiring. It's usually when a horse has been run down, when his stamina is exhausted, that he injures himself by taking a misstep over a jump.

"This was about a year ago. As a result of what was happening with their horses, some of my friends started taking it themselves just for the fun of it. Every one of them said how much they thought it increased their energy and stamina on long hunts. So I started taking it to see what would happen.

Sure enough, I noticed a difference in myself. Definitely more energy on 300 mg a day. But I think the best thing about it is the way it helps you recover from some insult to your body. Some time ago, I had a terrible accident with a horse and was quite badly hurt. While I was in the hospital, I was without my B-15's for several weeks, and when I was released I was just barely able to get around but still feeling a lot of discomfort. I got back on B-15 when I got home, and I'm convinced that all my injuries started to heal at double the rate they would have otherwise.''

Here we come to another significant claim made for B-15—that it promotes the healing of any component of the body that is damaged by inflammation caused by stress or trauma. This pertains particularly to athletic injuries, and numerous athletes, professionals, and weekenders alike have declared B-15 a magic remedy. For instance, Arthur Goldbeck, an avid weekend tennis player living in South Bend, Indiana, insists that B-15 cured him of a chronic leg muscle condition that had kept him off the courts for months. ''It first started about two years ago when I was playing in a singles tournament at my club. I learned that I had in my leg a muscle that I never knew about before. The reason I learned this was because I pulled the muscle—ruptured it, actually—when I was lunging to make a difficult volley. Suddenly my right leg—the leg I was pushing off—felt like it had been pierced by a high-caliber bullet. It collapsed on me and I fell in a heap of screaming pain on the court. Everyone was sure that I had fractured or broken my leg bone. But then a doctor was summoned from the clubhouse and he told me what it was. I had ruptured my plantaris muscle. The plantaris muscle is that muscle deep inside your calf that enables you to push off when you're walking or running. Well, I hadn't warmed up properly and the first time in the match when I had to push off and make an extra effort, the muscle snapped. It left me an absolute cripple for two weeks, and it was another two months before I could walk normally again. And that was with daily deep-heat treatments. Finally, after another month or so, I was able to play tennis again. So I went out and wouldn't you know, the first time I played the bloody thing snapped on me again! This time I knew what it was, and since then I've become an expert on the plantaris muscle. It happened two more times after that and it became like a chronic condition. I finally had to give up playing singles and stick to doubles, where I wouldn't have to extend myself so much.

"But then, I was on a combined vacation-business trip in Palm Springs eight months ago and was invited to play singles at the Palm Springs Racquet Club. Since I was trying to impress a potential business customer, I threw caution to the winds. I went at our match like Rod Laver and the inevitable happened. Midway through the third set, my leg exploded again. As it happened, a guy who was playing on an adjoining court was a doctor from L.A. Afterwards, in the locker room, we got talking. I told him all about the plantaris muscle, all the things I had learned about it, and of course he knew exactly what I was talking about. I told him my history—how it first went, and how it kept going over and over again. He suggested I try B-15. He described how the muscle was obviously in a chronically weakened condition as a result of the first episode and how it had never had a chance to heal properly because of the likelihood of impaired or lesser than desirable blood circulation to my lower extremities that affects men my age. To make a long story short, I got some of this B-15 and started taking it. I was that desperate. And I'll tell you what. Not only did my leg heal much faster than it ever had before—and by faster I mean the pain was gone within a week instead of two to three weeks and I was able to walk normally much sooner—but I've gone back to playing my all-out singles tennis without a recurrence of the injury. Since I started taking B-15, I haven't even had a twitch. In addition to that, I feel terrific all over and can play tennis longer and harder than I have in years. And you're talking to a man who is about to celebrate his sixty-fifth birthday."

Almost anyone who has watched professional football regularly, whether in a stadium or on television, has seen the following: A back or wide receiver is sprinting downfield to catch up with a perfectly thrown pass. The vectors seem ideal; the trajectory of the spinning ball and the course of the speeding, in-the-clear receiver are about to merge into what is a sure touchdown. But then, as the receiver raises his arm to gather in the ball, he staggers and falls, skidding ignominiously across the turf as the ball bounces harmlessly and he, gripping his thigh, writhes in some inexplicable agony.

What has happened is that in making that little extra effort to snare the football, the receiver has ruptured his hamstring muscle. The hamstring is the long, dense muscle that runs from the back of the thigh and over the rear of the knee to connect to the calf, and its purpose is to assist in the extension of the leg during walking and running. It is also a function of the hamstring to prevent hyperextension, or the collapsing of the knee joint rearward when the leg is extended to its fullest. During extraordinary effort or as a result of extraordinary extensor straining of the leg, the fibrous density of the hamstring will not be sufficient to prevent such hyperextension. Rupture—the sudden pulling apart of the muscle's fibers, which are cellular in composition like everything else in the body—occurs as a consequence.

The "pulled" or ruptured hamstring muscle is an affliction common to athletes who compete in hard-running sports. Track and field sprinters, football receivers, and baseball outfielders are particularly susceptible to hamstring pulls. Anthony Morelia, a trainer for the U.S. Olympic track team in 1976, tells of an experiment conducted by several medical nutritionists and sports medicine specialists during the past year among sprinters from several dozen colleges across the country. In the spring of 1978, 27 sprinters on the track teams of these colleges suffered severe hamstring pulls. The usual treatment of such injuries is a short rest, followed by various therapy applications such as ultrasound and deep-heat, massage, and whirlpool baths. Half the crippled athletes were given the usual treatment, while the other half were treated with nothing but a daily regimen of B-15 tablets in combination with Vitamins A and E. It was found, says Morelia, that the runners on B-15 were able to resume training almost a full week sooner than those on the conventional treatments. "It sort of confirmed the theory," he says, "that B-15 promotes increased oxygen to damaged cells and tissues and thereby hastens the healing process." Morelia adds that B-15 has become a staple in the medicine kits of trainers in the big-time football leagues, professional and collegiate. "Every one of them that I know is convinced the stuff definitely enhances the healing of all those nagging injuries that put players down for weeks on end. I have seen sore-armed baseball pitchers come back much sooner on B-15 than they otherwise would, and guys with serious sprains, jammed fingers, bad bruises, and charley horses—they all benefit from it."

Irv Rosenberg, a consultant to the Washington Redskins under George Allen, also stresses B-15's ability to speed healing. "That hamstring muscle ruptures very often in athletes," he notes. "I myself have ruptured it twice. But with B-15, I was out on the field again within 72 hours, whereas usually the treatment is ten days in a cast. Another player with the same injury got out there again in four days. I told a podiatrist about what a help B-15 had been, and he told me I should keep it to myself because it could put him out of business!"

How about the ordinary person who isn't trying for the All-American team or the Olympic world record, but just wants to increase his overall energy level? Here, too, B-15 enjoys a large and enthusiastic following. Although here too the reports are far from unanimous, one gets a generally favorable impression from interviewing people who use or have used B-15. Most respondents attribute all sorts of good things in their lives to pangamate, from increased stamina to more buoyant spirits and greater self-confidence.

It would certainly fit with the general theory as to B-15's effects on body metabolism that it should have psychological effects as well as physical ones. The general theory, of course, is that B-15 increases bloodstream and cell oxygenation, which in turn increases overall energy production in the body. It seems almost inevitable that this will raise the user's spirits as well. "I have seen clear-cut examples of increased personal courage and self-confidence in people who are regular users of B-15," says a San Francisco medical nutritionist and immunologist. "I myself find it easier to face up to ticklish situations in my life since I've been taking B-15, situations that I might well have shrunk from before. I find that I ski with less fear and am willing to tackle steeper slopes without my stomach getting tied up in knots, and that the terrible claustrophobia I used to have in elevators and such is now just a mild anxiety. I attribute this to the vastly increased energy I have from B-15. In my mind, energy is the arbiter and shaper of one's morale. The better you feel, the more energized and lively—even daring—you feel spiritually."

Dr. Robert Atkins echoes this view. He claims that B-15 "can turn a patient's energy picture around rather surprisingly." Moreover, he depends on B-15 himself. "If I forget to take it, I feel it. If I'm getting tired during the day and I have a meeting at night, I take three B-15 pills and I'm no longer tired." Atkins also believes that an individual's spiritual well-being—his self-confidence, his willingness to assert himself, his proclivity to get the most out of life unshackled by interior fears and anxieties—is a function of his energy level. "You seldom see high-energy people who are shrinking violets or who suffer from uncertain self-images. High-energy folks take more risks and are less prone to the negative psychological ramifications of rejection or failure. Whereas low-energy people are those you often see who have psychological problems—who suffer from depressions and psychological blockages. I wouldn't go so far as to say there is a clear-cut cause-and-effect relationship between psychological dysfunction and physiological energy function. But it's certainly a notion worth looking into more closely."

Many of the people one meets who are taking B-15 started on it because they had heard of its energy-boosting properties and of its reported ability to improve morale and reduce anxiety. As always, in the absence of scientifically controlled experiments, it is difficult to impossible to gauge the extent of the placebo effect in their reports; but the fact remains that many of them report some remarkable effects, even in circumstances when they began taking B-15 without any expectation of benefit—sometimes without any idea of what they expected to happen.

Marcia Melchionni, a divorced mother of three living in Washington, D.C., began suspecting that her oldest son was using drugs when he was a senior in high school. His personality had suddenly become so much more spirited that she felt sure he must be dabbling with chemical stimulants—uppers and downers, as she had heard them described. In fact, he was not using drugs but was taking B-15 tablets on a daily basis on the recommendation of his basketball coach; but being at the age when he shared nothing with his mother and resented any inquiries into his personal life as unwarranted meddling, he had not told her about it.

One day, Marcia's son left an almost full bottle of B-15 tablets stashed between the mattress and box spring of his bed and apparently forgot they were there. A few weeks later, Marcia found the bottle—its almost homemade-looking, plain label describing the contents as Aangamik-15—while turning the mattress of the bed. Her suspicions were confirmed. She hid the bottle and waited a few weeks for some indication from her son that he had missed it. When none came, she grew curious. Finally, Marcia's curiosity got the better of her and she decided to take one of the tablets to see "what kind of druggy reaction it had, so I could learn what in God's name kind of thrills Victor was getting from them."

Marcia swallowed one tablet and waited for the world to go into the kind of kaleidoscopic jumble she had heard certain drugs induced. Nothing happened. The next day, she swallowed two tablets. Still nothing. "I went on like this for several days, growing more and more mystified," she says. "I was getting no reaction whatsoever that I could tell until about the second week, when I took six tablets at one time. Then I felt something, but it was nothing like I expected—just a slight flushing of the skin that lasted maybe a minute. But after that, and for the next week, as I took more and more pills each day, I did notice something else. I had more energy. It used to be in the mornings after I got the kids sent off to school, I would lie down for a while and watch television and maybe grab a quick nap before lunchtime. Now I didn't want to do that. I had no patience for TV and I was jumping out of my skin to do something. After about a month, until Vic's bottle of pills was empty, I became a whirling dervish. I started doing exercises, walking the streets and parks of the city, going to museums, getting out of the house for long stretches every day where before I had never had the energy to get anything organized. And when I'd come home after a day out, I would still be full of pep and I'd make the kids these big Italian dinners, where before I was feeding them frozen lasagnas and stuff like that. And another thing, I'd always had insomnia, and now that completely disappeared.''

After the pills were exhausted, Marcia rapidly reverted to her previous sluggishness. ''By then, I knew it was the pills that were responsible, but I still thought they were some kind of dope. I didn't know how to get any more and I didn't dare ask Victor about them. I racked my brains trying to figure out a way to get more, but I assumed they were the kind of things you had to go out into back alleys at night in the rougher sections of town to buy, and I wasn't about to do that. I went for two months without them and fell completely back into my old ways. You know, little energy, little ambition. Then I happened to go to the basketball awards dinner at Victor's high school. The coach got up to speak and he started thanking everybody—the parents who supplied him with such talented boys, the teachers who let the boys off early for basketball practice, and so on and so on. And then, sort of whimsically, he held up a bottle of the same pills I had found, the Aangamiks. The team had been undefeated and he said, 'And last but not least, we owe a debt of gratitude to these little pills,' or something like that. I nearly fainted, thinking that he was pushing dope or something, and I thought all the parents would charge the dais and beat him to a pulp. But he went on to explain what they really were: vitamin pills that did such-and-such to your bloodstream and increased your energy and stamina. He was really giving his little lecture because one of the parents of the boys on the team was with the FDA and he was sort of saying it all for his benefit—you know, like, hey, why don't you fellows over there sharpen up to the fact that this stuff is okay? Anyway, I went up to him after the dinner and asked where I could get some. He told me it was available at any health food store. So I went to one and stocked up. And my life has been heaven ever since. Now we all take it openly—Victor and my other two kids—and we all have a good laugh about my suspicions."

Marvin Grosswirth, who authored two excellent articles on B-15 in *Science Digest* in the fall of 1978, testified in the first of them to his own experience with B-15. He deliberately picked a time when he knew that considerable demands would be made on his stamina. He began taking four tablets a day on a Tuesday morning and put in a ten-hour workday with hardly any trouble. The next day, he says, he left for a national convention of an organization for which he served as public relations officer. He had a grueling schedule, including a couple of speeches, several appearances on radio and TV, meetings, late-night parties, and if he was lucky maybe four hours' sleep each night. By Thursday, he reported, he was taking two extra tablets as a pick-me-up at about dinner time, and once he did that, the B-15 seemed to live up to its advance notice. "This was not the first such convention I had attended," he stated, "nor was it any easier than previous ones; indeed, in some ways, it was more demanding. Nevertheless, my spirits and stamina were unflagging, from early morning until late at night. After I returned home on Sunday, instead of experiencing the usual post-convention letdown, I was eager to begin work early the next morning. As for side effects, I felt only one: I was sleeping less, even when I wanted to stay in bed.''[1]

A world-famous entertainer writes to Da Vinci Laboratories about how their version of B-15 fuels his already impressive dynamo. "I have found it to be a remarkable source of energy for me," he writes in a bold, swift hand fairly bursting with vitality. "I usually do two shows a night working in Las Vegas. I take two 15's about an hour before I go on and I get through the night without one huff or puff. I swear it's even made me funnier!"

But the chorus of acclaim is far from unanimous. Dr. Victor Herbert, chief of the hematology and nutrition laboratory at the Bronx Veterans Administration Hospital and professor of medicine at the State University of New York, denounces claims of improvement resulting from B-15. "Every quack is going to have 80 percent satisfied customers," he declared in an interview for *Science Digest*, "because in 80 percent of all cases, whatever ailment brought the patient to [a] doctor or [to] a quack disappears within two weeks. Whatever they took or didn't take, whatever alteration they made in their diet or in their breathing or in their love life, will get the credit."

Dr. Robert Atkins, however, snorts derisively at this assertion. "People come to me complaining of fatigue," he declares, noting that he's treated about 500 people by now for this problem. "Each has been to six doctors on the average. Not one of those doctors was ever able to achieve a placebo-effect success yet . . . and then I give them B-15 and the patients say, 'What did you give me? I don't know what happened but I never felt better in my life!' It doesn't happen all the time. But it happens in about half the cases, and that's often enough to convince me that it is efficacious."

But the fact remains that some people do indeed find that B-15 does nothing much whatever for them. Professional basketball player Julius Erving noted no improvement in his already gifted performance or endurance after trying pangamate

[1] "B-15: Is It Superpill?" *Science Digest,* September 1978, p. 13.

for two months in 1977. Nor did aging star John Havlicek of the Boston Celtics, who tried it in an attempt to stem the waning tide of his stamina. Rod Gilbert, long a standout with the New York Rangers hockey team, took it for a while in an attempt to forestall forced retirement and found that it made no difference. Lesser lights in the sports world have also reported unencouraging results, while Sid Moret, a trainer for the New York Giants football team, calls B-15 "hogwash."

"We began hearing about B-15 three or four years ago, about how it brought about faster healing, and how it gave athletes more staying power and made them stronger. We tried it on some of the boys and I can tell you it made absolutely no difference. A lot of other trainers around the league had a shot at it too. If it's being used today with any regularity in the National Football League, then it's the best-kept secret in creation."

Bob Narcessian, director of the American Sports Medical Training Center, is dubious about B-15, too. "I think it's more gimmickry than anything else," he says. "One or two athletes I know have taken it, but I didn't see any tremendous changes in their performance. Some might say they felt better—and I've heard some say that—but I never saw anything that would convince me it was anything special."

Some even report adverse results from taking B-15. A particularly odd effect was reported by a prominent, world-class professional Australian tennis player, who started supplementing his diet with B-15 about two months before the Wimbledon tennis championships in June 1977. "A lot of the players on the tour had gotten into it and were giving it credit for all sorts of improvement in their endurance and energy. I figured that if it was that good and they were taking it, I'd better start taking it too or I would lose an advantage. So I started taking it—six, eight, ten pills a day—and, at first, I thought I noticed a difference. I could go longer in a tough set without tiring and losing my concentration, and I seemed to be able to explode the ball harder off my racket, putting more pace than ever on my ground strokes. But now, in retrospect, I wonder if that wasn't my imagination, something that I imagined was happening because I'd been led to believe it was supposed to happen. Certainly, I thought I felt better, but in the end my game didn't improve. After I was on it for about three months, I decided to quit. Well, that was a revelation. As soon as I got off it, my game went to hell. I was playing like a zombie—no energy, no power at all. So I went back on it, and my game gradually went back to normal. But it never got any better. I went off it again at the beginning of this year [1978] and the same thing happened. I began to feel drained again, tired all the time. I figured, Jesus, this is a strange pill—it doesn't really make you feel any better or give you more energy or improve your game, but once you stop taking it you go to pieces. A lot of the other guys experienced the same thing. So it must be doing something inside your system. I finally got off it for good because it scared me—the withdrawal effects. Once I decided to stop for good, it took me a good three months to get back to the energy level I'd always had.''

An enthusiastic amateur tennis player reports a similar effect. ''During the summer,'' he says, ''it's my custom to play three or four times a week, usually against players who are my equal or better, usually singles, and usually three to five sets at a time. The weather is invariably hot, and in recent years I had begun to notice that as I approached my mid-forties (I'm also a smoker), my energy flagged after two or three hard-played sets, robbing me of my concentration and competitive resolve. After two months on B-15, there seemed to be little if any improvement in my endurance. Nor did the power or pace of my shots materially benefit. Clearly, if I was to hope for increased stamina in this often physically furious sport, I would have had to quit smoking. By no measurable means did B-15 consumption counter the oxygen-reducing effects of my smoking habit.

''But I did experience something unexpected. Once I stopped taking B-15 pills on a daily basis, I noted a radical flagging of my normal energy levels. Where once, prior to

B-15, I was able to go through a day without ever feeling tired or dopey, I found myself sagging in the late afternoons. This lasted for about two weeks, and then my energy level returned to its normal state.''

What might explain such an effect? A lot of these individuals failed to say which version of B-15 they had been taking. Perhaps if they had, it would have shed some light on the puzzling variations in the results they reported. Another possibility might be that the difficulties some of these B-15 users reported were psychosomatic. But when queried, several doctors said no. They suggested that daily usage of B-15 had provided an increase of oxygen in the blood. These tennis players' systems had become accustomed to the increase, so that when they stopped B-15 their bodies rebelled. Cells that had benefited from enhanced respiration were suddenly crying out in oxygen hunger. It took them a good two weeks before they were able to readjust to the reduced oxygen they had been used to before.

One doctor explains the diversity of reaction thus: ''You've got to understand that different organisms react in different ways to pangamic acid—or, for that matter, to any other substance. For some, endurance is not a significant factor in their performance. Many athletes have higher natural levels of energy than others, and this all comes about through 'oxygen transfer'; that is, the ability of the body to transfer oxygen from sites where it's not needed to sites where it is. This has never really been studied, but I think it's accurate to say that certain people store oxygen better than others. It is the people who naturally don't store oxygen well that pangamate benefits most, in whom the differences are most clearly apparent in such things as endurance and stamina. I'm talking now about trained athletes, people who are already in good physical shape, who don't smoke or indulge in other oxygen-diminishing habits. These people are still different from each other in their natural ability to transfer oxygen. Some people have what you might call a natural reserve fuel tank, whereas others don't. Now the same thing exists with ordinary people, and the effects of B-15—the palpable effects—will be different among them as well. Two poorly oxygenated people who are equally out of shape will react differently to B-15 simply because one is naturally able to draw sooner on reserves than the other. It has a lot to do with their basic metabolisms.''

Well then, there's another area of vast ignorance: the differences among basic human metabolisms. Doctors who use nutritional therapies with their patients have many tales to tell about the unpredictable nature of the human metabolism and its sometimes capricious reactions to various substances. We have barely scratched the surface of our ignorance regarding the interrelationship of health, nutrition, and disease, and no matter which way we turn, we find more questions than answers. Certainly that is true in the whole controversy over B-15. Some people report marvelous results; others report nothing. *Something* happened to both groups—but what? And why? The truth is that we simply don't know as yet, and it's going to take a lot of careful investigation and research before we do. Meanwhile, sports and stamina are far from the only fields in which we hear reports of B-15's benefits. Another is that perennial and ever-fascinating topic: sex.

4

The Vitamin
With Sex Appeal

One topic you know is going to get people's attention is sex. Lecture them about nutrition, and they may be bored stiff. Suggest that their life style could be dangerous to their health and they may turn you off instantaneously. They may think sports and exercise are strictly for Phys. Ed. majors. But suggest that something can help their sex life and they are suddenly all ears. Thus, when reports began spreading that B-15 could do good things for you in bed, a lot of people started listening up in a hurry.

And no wonder. Some of the reports are pretty sizzling. Increased endurance. More brilliant climaxes. More frequent orgasms. Increased desire. It sounds like a sex manual and a wish book combined. No wonder people who couldn't care less about nutrition and preventive medicine have turned on to B-15 since hearing of its reported capacity to light up their sex life. Of the 62 current or former regular B-15 users interviewed for this book who were between the ages of 30 and 50, slightly more than 60 percent credited the substance with a measurable improvement in the quality of their sexual experience. Sexual excitation was easier to achieve, they reported, pleasure was more intense, and performance more fulfilling—that is, the men were able to perform longer while the women were able to reach orgasm sooner and/or experience more than one orgasm during a single incidence of intercourse. Of the remaining 38 percent, about half claimed to have undergone a marked increase in overall vitality and energy that may have resulted in enriched sexual enjoyment, although few were willing to attribute that enrichment solely to B-15, since most consumed the substance in combination with other nutritional energy supplements such as the B-Complex vitamins.

If B-15's manufacturers were allowed to make therapeutic claims for their product, these interviews would make dandy endorsements, although some of them would have to be X-rated. Take Martin Rappoport, for example, a 42-year-old producer of television commercials for a high-powered New York advertising agency. Until two years ago, before he started taking B-15 regularly in the form of calcium pangamate tablets after learning about it during a visit to California, he was the standard run-down, anxiety-ridden New York sophisticate who resorted to such stimulants as cocaine, hashish, and marijuana for the highs in his life. "Now," Martin says, "my whole life is a natural high. Since I've been using B-15, I no longer go through mood swings, ups-and-downs. My energy level is at least 50 percent higher on a sustained basis from the time I get up in the morning until I go to bed at night. I think more clearly, am more decisive, and just feel terrifically self-confident. If you had known the *old* me, you would have seen a guy walking on eggs all the time. Before B-15, I was Marty Rappoport, a guy who sort of shlumped through life and got little enjoyment from it. Now, I strut and stroll, and most of the time I feel as if I've got the world on a string."

What was the biggest change in Martin Rappoport's life that he attributed to B-15? "For several years, I took Vitamin E in the expectation that it would build up my sexual staying power. You see, that was always a problem with me, particularly after women started getting liberated and demanded more than just wham-bam-thank-you-ma'am. I found that I couldn't cut the mustard with a lot of women back in the early seventies. So I got into E, but it didn't make any difference. Then I found B-15. After two months on six tabs a day, I noticed I could go all night. And it's gotten better ever since."

What a sensation, then, in a society that has become so obsessed with sexual performance. Is B-15 about to displace power as the ultimate aphrodisiac? To hear some people talk, you might think it already has. Take Don Shaffer, a married college-alumni fund raiser in his mid-thirties, who said that after three months of B-15 usage his sexual experience quadrupled in the joy and intensity of its pleasure, which in turn vastly increased his overall sense of psychological well-being. "Not that it has increased my biological sex drive per se," he explains. "But the quality of my orgasms has expanded and improved immensely, and that in itself has increased my sex drive. Believe me, when I started taking B-15, I never thought of it in terms of sex. I was merely trying it out because I'd heard it provided more energy and I was finding myself sagging toward the end of the day at the office. But it had this almost immediate effect of cranking up my sexual capacity.

"The better sex began to get, the more I wanted it. My wife and I had gone through Masters and Johnson-type therapies and other kinds of counseling five and six years ago when our sex life went stale and I became sort of impotent due to my anxiety over her failure to have orgasms. Then we went through Vitamin E and other nutrition kicks—to no avail. About a year ago, we started on B-15, and I'll tell you, it has turned our sex lives around. Can you imagine the feeling, after being married twelve years, to suddenly find your wife a terrific turn-on again? And not only that, but to realize that she feels the same way about you? Where she and I had settled into a once or twice a month schedule until last year, we now go at it four, five, sometimes six times a week—sometimes three or four times a night. And it's not just me, it's her too. Suddenly she's having orgasms like crazy and wants sex just as much as I do. She's always ready, and it's practically saved our marriage."

Debbie Shaffer confirms Don's claims. "Our problem was

that it took me ages to have an orgasm, and Don just couldn't keep going long enough to bring me off. As a result, I began to feel deprived and then secretly resentful. I lost interest in sex and found that I could live very well without it. I did have an affair once, though, which Don knows about. He was a wonderful older guy and was able to maintain control long enough to occasionally bring me to orgasm. After it was over, I went back to Don and got him into sex therapy because my affair had reawakened my libido. We had only partial success from that. Then, after trying a lot of other things, we discovered B-15 and it has changed our lives radically for the better. We didn't get into B-15 with sex in mind, but that's really turned out to be the bottom line of it. Now Don can last longer, and at the same time it doesn't take me so long to reach orgasm—ten to fifteen minutes as compared to an hour or more previously. We have reached a happy, delicious medium, and for the first time since the beginning of our marriage, I'm really in love again with my husband. I could never think of looking for someone else, as I once did.''

Similar testimonials abound to the sexual-improvement effects of pangamic acid from mainly monogamous, heterosexual married couples. Even more enthusiastic were several people who led more varied and diverse sex lives. One, Bill Boyd, a twice-divorced bachelor, had had trouble for several years enjoying his sexual freedom. "After my second divorce, I vowed never to marry again, but just to get the most out of life that I could, romantically, emotionally, sexually. Both my marriages broke up principally because of lousy sex, and I figured I had a lot of catching up to do. I had determined that staying with one partner for a lot of years was death to any relationship—there's just no way you can stay sexually interested in her, or her in you. So I went out, and, sure enough, I found plenty of free, varied, and if I may say so, wild sex to be had. But much to my dismay, I couldn't perform, or could just barely perform. I learned through therapy that my old-fashioned 1950's values—you know, the man as the aggressor—were being threatened by the new and liberated attitudes of most of the women I encountered. It took only one or two of them telling me that I had been lousy in bed to turn me into a quivering, impotent, sex-fearing vegetable.

"I went on like that for a couple of years and then happened on B-15, learning about it from, of all people, a prostitute. Afterwards, maybe a month or so after starting a daily intake of calcium pangamate, I found myself in a situation with a girl where it was either fish or cut bait, either accept her invitation to go to bed with her or make up some excuse and leave. I gambled on fishing and it turned out to be great, a fantastic lay, even though I still felt intimidated by the girl's aggressiveness and abandon. A few more times with other such girls and I was cured. Intimidation was no longer a factor in my head. Suddenly I was a regular sex machine and was able to screw anything in skirts. Not only that, but my orgasms took a long time coming and were just mind-blowingly fantastic when they did. For years before, my orgasms at best—like when I was married—were ordinary and all centered in my penis, a quick ejaculatory thrill that passed as quickly as it arrived and was accompanied by a certain amount of. . .well, sadness. I had begun to think that I was simply getting old and that my prostate was beginning to give out on me. But now, my orgasms are invariably gigantic, sustained rushes that blast through by entire body. I lose complete control of myself and literally see stars. For twenty or thirty seconds, it's like I'm flying through space, and it even scares some of the women I've slept with. Man, you'll never catch me without B-15 again!"

Gwen Powers is a 32-year-old failed dress designer who decided to use her body as her principal source of income when her business collapsed several years ago. She became a $100-a-night call girl serving prosperous out-of-town businessmen visiting New York's poshest hotels. She had no qualms about her new trade but found the often thrice-a-night sex she engaged in an increasingly unsettling source of boredom and dispiritedness. Then she discovered B-15. Bill Boyd was not a client but a friend, and it was she who introduced him to the idea of taking B-15 for his sexual problem.

"I started using pangamate along with other vitamins on a doctor's orders after a bout with hepatitis and gonorrhea," Gwen reports. "Within weeks, a curious change came over me. I started enjoying the paid sex I was having, no matter who I was having it with, became hornier than hell, and began to have orgasms with some of my more proficient clients. At first, I didn't know what to ascribe it to, I sure as hell didn't know what B-15 was—it was just another of the dozens of pills and tablets I was taking during the day.

"After a couple of weeks, my supplies ran out—the B-15 and the other vitamins—and I began to revert to my former boredom about sex. It became routine again, pure work, no enjoyment from the act. One night, I was in a client's bathroom at the Sherry Netherland Hotel and looked inside the medicine cabinet. There was a bottle of calcium pangamate. I recognized it from the collection of various bottles I had had when I was taking vitamins during the previous months. For some reason, I decided to swipe it. I put it in my bag, took it home with me, and started swallowing four or five pills a day. I still didn't know anything about it and made no connection between it and the sexual enjoyment I had experienced earlier. Within a week, I started to get turned on again by the sex I was having. By turned on, I mean I was having orgasms with almost every guy who put his cock inside me, as long as he could last a few minutes. The bottle of B-15 pills ran out after two weeks, but by that time I was a sexual dervish—really enjoying my work, so to speak. Some nights, I would even go out looking for free sex.

"But once the bottle had run out, I went back to the old boredom again. That's when I made the connection between B-15 and sexual pleasure. I went and bought another bottle at a health food store and bang! it all began to come back again. I haven't stopped using it since."

Enough of the interviewees for this book noted such a

perceptible or radical improvement in sexuality that it seemed appropriate to consult several doctors for an explanation of the possible physiological and biochemical reasons why.

Several physicians debunked the likelihood of any direct biochemical cause-and-effect relationship between B-15 consumption and better sex, attributing the phenomenon solely to human psychology. One, for example, said, "Listen, I've seen it happen a thousand times. You give somebody a sugar-coated pill, tell him it's a painkiller and will relieve his pain, and nine times out of ten he'll call you a few hours later and say that the pain has disappeared. These people who are taking this B-15 have been led to believe it will make sex more terrific for them. So they take it and sex gets more terrific. Read Freud on the power of suggestion. Or read any good psychology text on self-fulfilling prophecy. It's strictly the placebo effect.

"Even if B-15 is useful in the treatment of certain diseases, and I'm not saying it is, there's no reason to believe that it's going to have an effect on sexuality in any physiological or biochemical sense. Sexuality is all in the mind, anyway. Who was it that said that the most potent sex organ is the brain? If you're in the mood and everything else is right and you're feeling good about yourself and your partner, then you'll have good sex. If there's something nagging at you below the surface of your conscious, it's likely to be not so good. Most people always have something nagging at them. Sometimes they are able to transcend it when they get into sex, but most of the time they can't. And when they can't, sex is not as terrific as it is on the occasions when they can.

"That's the suggestive power of something like B-15. Someone starts taking it and the fact that he's taking it for the purpose of achieving more sexual energy, staying power, or whatever occupies his subconscious and temporarily drives out whatever it is that usually nags at him. So he performs or enjoys better than usual. And then he attributes it to the chemical effects of B-15, rather than to the fact that the positive conceptual suggestion of B-15—that it will improve his sex—has nudged aside his usual anxieties. Taking B-15 for sexual purposes is nothing more than an exercise in self-hypnosis. Terrific if it works. But I could give you an M & M candy, tell you it was a potent, instant-acting, six-hour sexual stimulant that would enable you to perform as you never have before, and for the next six hours you would be carrying on like Casanova. That's an exaggeration, but you get my point. It's all in the mind.''

Well, undeniably, suggestion *could* have something to do with it, but not everybody is so totally suggestible as this doctor seemed to assume. Moreover, how about the people like Gwen Powers who had no notion when they began taking B-15 that it would do anything at all for their sex lives? And she isn't alone. A number of other interviewees insisted that when they began taking B-15 they had no thoughts in their minds that it would improve their sexuality. Energy, yes, but not their ability to perform sexually to greater emotional or sensory profit. How can those skeptical physicians explain this?

"If B-15 does increase the energy level when taken on a regular basis," said another doctor, "then it's perfectly conceivable that it will improve sexual function and all the things that go with it. Because sex is so important to so many people, those who find an increase in their overall energy levels as a result of B-15 consumption would be likely to note that increase particularly in their sexual functioning. And then they say, 'Ha! Sex is getting better, so this B-15 must be an aphrodisiac of some sort.' The fact is that sex is a function of energy. The more energy you have, the better you are likely to perform at any physical activity. Sex is the kind of physical activity that most people take particular notice of. By that I mean how they perform, how long they can last, how much pleasure they get out of it. A typist working in an office might notice, after taking B-15 or any other energy booster for a while, that she can type longer without fatigue, without getting a backache, without growing bored, and so on. Since this is basically a mechanical activity, she won't get any particular thrill out of it, she'll probably just say 'how nice.' But sex for most of us is not rote but something special and everybody wants to be good at it and has lots of anxieties over it. So if this typist's sexual experience improves along with her typing experience, she'll not just say 'how nice' but will tend to exult in it. Wouldn't you?''

Other doctors I talked to—urologists, endocrinologists, gynecologists, internists, and psychiatrists—were not so quick to dismiss the role of B-15 in sexual function as mind over matter. Two, in fact, gave similarly exhaustive, if speculative, explanations of how and why pangamic acid consumption may have a direct physiological effect on improved sexual function. According to one, an endocrinologist who marginally supports certain of the medicinal claims made for B-15, ''We can be reasonably sure from what little research has been done that B-15 most likely promotes increased oxygenation of the circulatory system, providing a corresponding infusion of greater amounts of oxygen into the cells and tissues of the body. If you look at the human sexual organs, male and female, you will see them basically as muscles made up of cells and tissues fed and nourished by veins and capillaries and energized by the nervous system. In moments of sexual excitation, the sexual organs of both men and women become engorged with blood, causing tumescence and involuntary pulsation in the man and expansion, lubrication, and pulsation in the woman. Remember also that the female clitoris is a cell-tissue muscle and that it too expands or becomes tumescent through blood engorgement as a result of sexual excitation.

''Under ordinary circumstances with the average man or woman, the blood that engorges the sexual organs during excitation is normally or subnormally oxygenated, depending on their general states of health, age, and so on. In other words, the blood is sufficiently oxygenated to enable basic engorgement, copulation, and ejaculatory completion to take place. Nature did not devise the copulatory process with a consideration for the pleasure, not to mention extended pleasure, the participants might get out of it. Nature devised intercourse solely for the purpose of procreation. The pleasure factor or pleasure demand has been evolved and added on by humans. And the extended-pleasure factor—you know, the long, leading-up-to-the-gigantic-orgasm process—has merely been a human refinement of this, something to be desired and pursued now that, in our human evolution, we no longer think of sex purely in procreative terms, as one does with other animals.

"You see, then, that although men and women seek prolonged, heightened sex, they do not yet have the natural biochemical tools to achieve it. Their organs, hormonal systems, and so on are still in the Stone Age, so to speak, still designed to function only for the purpose of procreation. Which means, to put it bluntly, that male-female physiology and neurology provide only the basic necessities for whatever pleasure accompanies the procreative process. The rest is up to human psychology. Human psychology has a great deal to do with the pleasure to be gotten from sexual coupling. More and more lately, pleasure has been defined by performance. In other words, the more capably two people are able to perform, the more pleasure they give and receive from the sex act.

"The emphasis on performance has brought about a concentration by men and women to consciously control the neuromechanical factors of the sex act. That is, the man, who is ordinarily quickly orgasmic by nature, is required to postpone his orgasm despite the neurological stimuli on his erect penis, and the woman, who is ordinarily slowly orgasmic, is required to speed up her orgasm time. The way couples have generally achieved this, or tried to, is through psychophysical techniques. But these techniques, though they may succeed occasionally, cannot be relied upon to work with unerring consistency. Indeed, preoccupation with them or excessive concentration on them often produce the opposite of the desired ends. Which is to say that the man will start 'prematurely' ejaculating or the woman will take longer and longer to reach orgasm.

"Now along comes something like B-15. With B-15 operating in the circulatory system at the times of sexual encounter and excitation, the sexual organs of the man and woman are not just engorged with blood in what have been normally oxygenated ways, they are engorged hypernormally—that is, their organs are receiving blood or filling with blood that contains much more oxygen than they are used to. This phenomenon can have scintillating effects. It can cause greater erections in men and more orgasm-sensitive reactions in the vaginas and clitorises of women. A penis with a greater than ordinary erection usually if not always is too 'hard' and therefore too insensitive to copulatory stimuli to achieve ejaculation. Therefore, the man suddenly finds himself able to delay his orgasm without even wanting to. Conversely, a greater blood engorgement of a woman's organs promotes in her a greater sensitivity to the stimulus of the man's superhard penis. As a consequence, she finds orgasm quicker and easier to arrive at, and may also enjoy the dividend of several orgasms while her lover's penis remains too hard for him to reach orgasm. Once the man has observed his partner experience one or more orgasms, this in itself will usually be so exciting to him that his penis will then relax enough to permit him to reach his own ejaculation-orgasm.

"It's through such a process that B-15 may very well have real as opposed to imaginary sexual benefits. By enabling the circulatory system to transport greater amounts of oxygen to the tissues of the sexual organs of men and women during times of sexual encounter—and by that I mean more oxygen than they are accustomed to—it permits the organs to function at optimum power. Not power in the sense of procreation, but power in the sense of pure muscle-nerve function. Many people, especially men, have long taken Vitamin E on the mistaken notion that E promotes virility and staying power. Vitamin B-15 may well be the substance that really provides the effects they thought or hoped they were getting from Vitamin E."

Another doctor, this one a urologist, compares the effects of B-15 on male sexuality to those of vasectomy and comes up with a similar conclusion. "We know," he says, "that after a man submits himself to a vasectomy,[1] his sexual prowess undergoes marked involuntary improvement insofar as controlling orgasm and ejaculation is concerned. Some of this may be psychological, of course. A man who has no anxiety about impregnating a woman may find that his pursuit of the pure pleasure of sex grows paramount. But it is in a much greater sense a physiological phenomenon. The man still manufactures sperm, but because it has no outlet, it is resorbed by the bloodstream. Within a short time, his hormonal, circulatory, and neurological systems adjust to the fact that they are no longer needed to manufacture and expel sperm through the penis. So they divert themselves to what can be considered the purely pleasurable aspects of copulation. The man still attains orgasm, he still ejaculates—though in lesser quantity—but he simply does not ejaculate sperm.

"With the task of producing and transporting the sperm removed, the blood-supply system and neurological networks concentrate solely on the feeding and nourishment of the erectile tissues in the penis. With these tissues getting more nourishment than they are accustomed to, they become more potent and are able to keep the penis erect for longer and longer periods—without ejaculation. Most men who undergo vasectomies are pleasantly surprised by this. There is no question that when an erection is extraordinarily hard and big the skin of the penis becomes stretched to its limits, and the neurological networks underneath become temporarily desensitized to the ordinary sensations of friction and warmth experienced inside a woman's vagina. This produces what most women would think of as enormous control on the man's part, although what they don't realize is that the man's 'performance' is largely involuntary—that he is holding off not so much because he wants to but because he cannot reach orgasm

---

[1] Vasectomy is the surgical method by which a man achieves sterility for birth-control purposes. The procedure consists of tying off or excising the vas deferens, the duct of the testis that carries sperm from the scrotum to the penis at times of erection and ejaculation.

as quickly as he might have before. He will attain orgasm, of course, but for some vasectomized men, it can take a bit of time, hours even. It is not for nothing that vasectomy, a man's operation, has been called the 'woman's operation' more and more lately as women's sexual pleasure has become the focus of so many people's attention.

"Vitamin B-15, assuming that it works in the manner it is said to, can take the place of a vasectomy for many men with regard to sexual performance or staying power. By increasing the oxygen uptake into the cells of the erectile tissues of the penis during intercourse, it can bring about larger and tauter erections, producing the same kind of temporary skin-and-nerve desensitization that produces such staying power. This is theory, mind you. Whether it in fact happens, or whether there is something else that occurs as a result of B-15 being introduced into the system, or whether nothing having to do with B-15 happens, no one knows for sure. But I too have heard a number of claims among my patients who are B-15 users that their sexual staying power has improved immensely. It is my guess that there's a direct biochemical and physiological link between oxygen-rich blood and erection intensity. Most men have 'tired' erections and ejaculate very quickly—just the work of getting the erection exhausts the oxygen in the blood supply to the penis, thereby exhausting the erectile tissue, oversensitizing the penis's nerves, and causing rapid ejaculations. The well-oxygenated penis, on the other hand, can undergo much more work and stress—just as any muscle can—before it grows tired and its nerves become sensitized. B-15, it is my conjecture, supplies that oxygenation. Which is why men on B-15 are suddenly finding themselves so adept at controlling their ejaculations. So sure am I of this that I have lately taken to recommending that certain patients of mine, aging men who have trouble getting or maintaining erections during intercourse, take B-15 regularly. It is too early to tell for sure, but preliminary reports from these patients indicate that it works to a large extent."

Sexual pleasure is not quite the absolute necessity of life

that physical health is, nor is something that does wonderful things for your sex life quite in the same league with something that can alleviate or perhaps prevent arteriosclerosis. But few people take seriously the possibility that they might get sick, or even die, before the hard reality presents itself to them, whereas a great many of us in this sex-conscious age think about our sex lives and ponder ways of improving it. The American public may or may not come to insist that its governmental regulatory agencies give B-15 a chance to prove its medicinal and therapeutic abilities, providing they hear enough stories about what B-15 has done for other people. But one cannot help wondering if it might not be B-15's reported ability to put pizzazz into your sex life that in the end foments the sort of popular pressure that may very well be needed if the FDA is ever to be budged.

Well, pizzazz certainly seems to be the story. ''I've had about 150 calls in the past year from doctors saying that guys who were impotent aren't impotent any more after about two weeks on B-15,'' says Dom Orlandi. Then he laughs and remembers a story. ''This guy had been on B-15 for about two weeks, and he called me up and said, 'Hey, will this stuff give you an erection?' I said, 'How would I know, I've never had a problem!' So then he told me that, about three o'clock that morning, he had gotten one so big it woke him up—and his wife thought she had a new toy! I told him I'd never heard of that one—although I sure have heard about it since that time. Then he stopped taking B-15, and his problem returned. And when he started taking it again, everything was fine. You can imagine he's taking it pretty regularly now!

''In fact,'' Dom Orlandi smiles, remembering still another story, ''there was one guy in Florida who had had a stroke that had left him unable to walk and pretty much knocked out his sex life, too. He started taking our B-15, and pretty soon he was walking without a cane, where before there hadn't been much hope for him.

''After he'd been on it for about two weeks, though, he noticed that things were happening in bed too. So he told us he wanted to become a distributor. He was going to call it 'Love Vitamins'! He ordered a whole consignment of B-15, and for a while he paid well, right on schedule. Then all of a sudden he wasn't paying on time.

"Well, a little while later, I was down in Florida on a visit, and just out of curiosity I did a little checking around, and I found out that he'd been going through two or three secretaries a week, because he'd always start chasing them! No wonder none of his bills got paid! He wasn't busy marketing at all—he was just popping all those 'Love Vitamins' himself and chasing all the young girls around!''

5

B-15
and Disease

Question: What do the following all have in common?

Alcoholism
Allergies
Arthritis
Asthma
Autism
Cardiovascular disease
Diabetes
Emphysema
Premature aging

Answer: They are all conditions that reportedly have been successfully treated using B-15.

The evidence is incomplete, of course, for all the reasons we've already gone into, notably the dearth of carefully designed, scientifically controlled experiments and the questions left unanswered by the Soviet studies. But, then, it is hard to see how the evidence could be anything *but* incomplete, inasmuch as the necessary research has been actively obstructed in this country by the United States government.

Consequently, the vast bulk of the evidence comes from the Soviet Union, although some pretty remarkable reports have accumulated from American sources, too. This evidence is arresting, to say the least, as we shall shortly see. Yet all too often the Soviet studies are dismissed out of hand by members of the American medical establishment and the governmental bureaucracy. In part, this is because of the problems we've already described arising from the differences in the Soviet and the American approaches to research and experimental design. But as one listens to the chorus of pooh-poohs from the American medical establishment, one begins to suspect that there is somehow more to it than just that.

All too often, one begins remembering, American scientists have seemed to succumb to an unwarranted superiority complex where Russian science is concerned, assuming that the Soviets must necessarily be behind us in any field of importance. Once upon a time, for example, we assumed that the Soviets could never work out the principles of atomic fission on their own—and then we explained their upsetting success in doing just that by convincing ourselves that they must have stolen the knowledge from us. Later, we largely ignored the potential of outer space until the Soviets successfully launched Sputnik—and then found ourselves deeply shocked by this trailblazing Soviet achievement. More recently, we have dismissed for some time the idea that the Russians may be approaching a breakthrough in the esoteric field of particle-beam weapons—"Buck Rogers" killer-ray guns that could knock missiles out of the sky—and now find ourselves confronted with disturbing evidence suggesting that the Soviets might indeed just be on to something there that could change every rule of the present East-West strategic arms balance.

Maybe it's time to revise our outlook.

That doesn't mean accepting the Soviet studies on B-15 uncritically. They *do* leave important questions unanswered, such as the precise chemical nature of the "calcium pangamate" that was used, and what B-15's clinical effects are alone, unassisted by other vitamins such as A and E. But can we honestly justify our steadfastly ignoring the amazing and hope-inspiring possibilities these studies suggest for ameliorating or even curing diseases that daily cause untold pain and grief to millions of human beings? Is it not at least worth investigating the matter for ourselves?

Take the first in that list of illnesses at the beginning of this chapter: alcoholism. If B-15 did no more than help in the treatment of this one affliction, it would still be worth close investigation. The Soviets, we know, have a special interest in alcoholism; for whatever problems our own society may have with this tragic ailment, they are mild compared to its ravages in the U.S.S.R. Uncounted workdays are lost as a result of it. Russian newspapers and periodicals constantly print articles decrying its effects on health, productivity, and the family. Indeed, alcohol abuse has deep roots in Russian history, where vodka served in Czarist times as the anodyne for the brutal, cheerless life of the serf, and where its influence continues today to the point that a defecting Soviet pilot complained because ground maintenance crews would on occasion drain the jet antifreeze from the aircraft's engines and drink it. (The pilot noted that this was a flying hazard never mentioned in the manuals.)

The Soviets concluded from their work with B-15 that it had great promise in treating chronic alcoholics. Moreover, it seemed to work in the most efficient way possible, not by suppressing symptoms but by eliminating the physiological addiction itself. Reporting on his work with 50 chronic alcoholics between 1961 and 1964, Dr. I. V. Strelchuk of the Central Research Institute of Forensic Psychiatry in Moscow found that B-15 brought about significant improvement in all of them. At the beginning of the experiment, the patients suffered from a pathological craving for drink. They were incapable of resisting alcohol. But all that changed after they had been treated with 80–100 milligrams of calcium pangamate a day for 20–30 days. They became indifferent to alcohol, he reported, even when they were exposed to the sight of a drink or were put into drinking company. He concluded that pangamate interrupted the chemical process in alcoholics that leads to their addiction, and thus eliminates their craving for alcohol. Even more arresting, Dr. Strelchuk concluded that "Vitamin B-15 has a particularly favorable effect in patients with chronic alcoholism accompanied by severe somatic changes. Cardiovascular diseases, hepatitis, and cirrhosis of the liver ceased progressing and then underwent regression toward a speedier restoration of the normal functions of the organ involved."

Well, 50 patients isn't an awful lot, and there *is* that recurrent problem of the absence of a control group. Dr. Strelchuk's findings are certainly intriguing. Still, we'd want to test them for ourselves before we really were convinced. But thus far no such research has been completed in the United States. Recently, a West Coast doctor did begin using B-15 to treat alcoholics and drug-abuse patients, and he was beginning to see some very encouraging results. Then he was forced to suspend his research when his neighbors, displeased that his work was bringing so many alcoholics and drug addicts into the neighborhood, pressured him to move. To date, he has been unable to find a suitable location for beginning again.

But evidence from other quarters has begun to trickle in. On the East Coast, Dr. Bernard Green, a New York City psychotherapist, has gotten excellent results using B-15 not only with alcoholism but with a whole list of other problems including arteriosclerosis, senility, hyperactivity, and emphysema. Indeed, talking to Dr. Green, who hails from Ireland originally, and studied with Adele Davis in his early years, will distinctly cheer up your day, for he can regale you with one case history after another in which some chronically ill person has found new life and health from a treatment prominently featuring B-15. Rarely these days do you find so many stories with happy endings.

For example, Dr. Green tells the story of Jim, a man in New York City with a twenty-five-year history of alcoholism. "Jim had had a serious drinking problem for years, but now it had gotten to the point where it was ruining his life. He had lost a big job as vice-president of a major New York firm because of his drinking, and it was breaking up his marriage, too. He came to me more or less as a last resort. I put him on daily doses of Vitamin E, niacinamide, and pantothenic acid, plus a breakfast drink heavy on brewer's yeast, lecithin, and protein. I also had him take 6 tablets of B-15 a day. After two months, his alcohol addiction had disappeared and he had quit drinking entirely—this after a quarter century of alcohol abuse! Today his marriage is back together, and he is back at his old firm once more as a vice-president.''

Why does Dr. Green think B-15 gets the results he has observed? ''I have my own private theory as to the origins of alcoholism,'' he answers. ''My theory is that most alcoholics have a basic low blood sugar, hypoglycemia problem, and their alcohol addiction results from the fact that they are addicted to sugar—alcohol, as you know, is converted into sugar in the bloodstream. B-15 normalizes blood sugar, and I think this is why it eliminates that uncontrollable craving for drink that makes somebody an alcoholic. I've used B-15 for years in treating alcoholism, first in Ireland, then later in Switzerland. I was also invited by the Polish government to give an address at Warsaw University on the subject. The Poles use B-15 extensively for this purpose, and with great success.''

A doctor who insists on total anonymity has been treating alcoholics with B-15 (in the form of DMG) at an alcoholic treatment center in the Northeast. He had 11 chronic drinkers, seven of whom were taking B-15. They were given quite a hefty dose—12 tablets a day—but they used nothing else, so this is one instance in which other nutritional substances do not cloud the issue. All seven were able to stop drinking completely. After ninety days the doctor found he could leave out in view any sort of liquor, even the patient's favorite kind, and trust the patient in the room alone with it, and he would never touch the stuff. As of this writing, these patients have been successfully off alcohol for six months. They are still taking B-15. The doctor considers B-15 an effective alternative to Antabuse, although he stresses that a necessary part of its success is the patient's desire to help himself. Some of the patients, moreover, had tissue samples taken from their livers to assess the degree of damage caused by the sclerosis of the liver that their drinking had brought on. The patients on B-15 found that the sclerosis was diminishing in size, and that their livers were beginning to regenerate.

FoodScience/Da Vinci Laboratories has several fat files of testimonial letters written to them over the years telling of the remarkable results that their B-15 (known as Aangamik-15 and Gluconic-15) has brought to often desperate people suffering a long list of maladies. One of these letters comes from a salesman on the West Coast. He says he is 41 years old and had long been a chronic alcoholic. "In September 1977," he writes, "I spent six weeks in a treatment center in a V.A. hospital in Tacoma, Washington, but I began drinking again soon after my release. I entered still another center in Montana in February 1978. I spent 28 days there, with strong support from Alcoholics Anonymous. After this, I remained sober, but lacking in real determination, ambition, or drive, my moods fluctuating wildly from highs to lows. Then in March 1978 I read the article in *New York Magazine* about B-15 and gave it a try, taking 150 mg a day. That was two months ago, and I'm amazed, simply amazed. I' VE TAKEN MY LAST DRINK. If the FDA wants proof, or is really interested in the welfare of the people of this country, they shouldn't turn their back on me. If there is any way I can be of help to you or your product, let me know."

From alcohol to allergies. The latter can range from insignificant to drastic in their effects. For some, they are no more than an annoyance—the itching of a mosquito bite, a stuffy nose from dust or ragweed or cats. But for others, they are life-crippling afflictions—swelling so severe from an insect bite that emergency antihistamine shots are needed to keep the victim from suffocating; asthma that threatens to make breathing impossible. A standard, effective treatment for allergic reactions is antihistamines. Several doctors who use B-15 in their work say that it seems to have an antihistamine-like effect. One reports his own experience. "I'm strongly allergic to garlic," says Dr. Howard Lutz of Washington,

D.C., "but I also like to try different cuisines, and my garlic allergy can limit that as you may well imagine. Well, one evening, we decided to try a new Thai restaurant in town. I knew that Thai cooking was pretty heavy on the garlic, and indeed, when we came into the place, you could smell it in the air. But I had decided to see what B-15 could do for me. So before we went, I had taken fifteen 50-mg tablets of B-15— and instead of my usual strong reaction, I had none at all! Not even a mild one!''

Dr. Lutz goes on to note some wider implications of B-15's potential in treating allergies. "Allergies do more than produce the sorts of reactions we all are familiar with; you know, the sneezing, or the swelling, or the rash. They can also lie at the root of excessive tiredness. I work mostly with people who come to me complaining of chronic fatigue. That means they wake up in the morning feeling tired after a full night's sleep. Or they feel suddenly tired after eating. It's also the 'stale athlete' syndrome. I have found that this problem is usually caused by undetected food allergies—you'd be amazed what odd things people can sometimes be allergic to! I put these people on a thoroughgoing nutritional program and I give them about 100–150 milligrams a day of B-15, although I will probably give an athlete about 300 milligrams a day, and sometimes as much as 3–5 grams, depending on his problem and his responsivenesss. I have been very pleased with the results I get this way. In fact, I'd go so far as to say that B-15 will get you good results in *all* conditions, because I've seen it do so many different things. I've used it with hyperactive children and seen their handwriting improve even after short periods of time on relatively modest dosages. I've seen it improve physical stamina quite markedly. It also works well with chelation therapy. And it seems especially useful for aged patients, almost rejuvenative in its effects.''

Some particularly striking evidence appears in an article by Dr. Allan Cott, a New York City psychiatrist who works extensively with children. In 1975 he published an article entitled "Pangamic Acid" in the *Journal of Orthomolecular Psy-*

chiatry which contained nine remarkable case histories of children suffering from hyperactivity, retardation, allergies, and asthma whose conditions had been dramatically improved by B-15. The case histories are in the form of letters from the children's parents. This renders them particularly poignant for the emotions they contain of relief and gratitude at having found help when all else had failed. Again, we must note that case histories and individual testimonials are not the same as controlled experiments capable of producing statistically significant results, but these case histories cannot be ignored, either, so eloquent and arresting are the cures they report.

The mother of a 10-year-old boy wrote about her son's long and agonizing history of violent allergies. Whenever he had been exposed to grasses, molds, ragweed, or other such pollen carriers, his breathing had become impaired to the point where he could hardly draw breath, and his eyes would also water and itch. Then he began taking B-15. His allergy problem dwindled to nearly nothing. To drive the point home, his mother wrote of how a period had come when his B-15 supply had run out and she had had trouble finding more. His allergies came back in force, and he had several attacks so severe that his doctor instructed her to begin bringing him in for more frequent treatments. But when he resumed taking B-15, his problems disappeared again. In a way, therefore, the boy acted as his own control group, inasmuch as his symptoms correlated closely to the times when he was taking B-15. Not a conclusive finding—but an extraordinarily promising one.

Another of Dr. Cott's case histories concerned an 11-year-old girl who suffered from severe hay fever. Writing in the summer, her mother told how she had begun giving her daughter B-15 six months earlier during the previous winter. She reported that it was the first summer in three years that her daughter had not had any hay fever. She also noted that the B-15 seemed to improve her daughter's mood and equanimity, reporting that "if she is without B-15 for more than a few days, her behavior changes and she is constantly angry. Whenever she does have the B-15, she is much more cooperative and alert.'' (This is yet another of B-15's areas of possible promise, as we shall see shortly in connection with the treatment of retarded or emotionally disturbed children.)

Other reports come from FoodScience/Da Vinci Laboratories' files. A Vermont man wrote with delight and gratitude about his wife's relief from a tenacious skin allergy. ''We heard of B-15 from a friend who had been taking it for several months,'' he relates. ''He looked so good, I asked him if he was taking some kind of magic pill, and he said, 'you hit it, that's exactly right.' My wife has had chronic skin trouble for years and has been to doctors, hospitals, etc., all over the United States without much success. Her condition is called eczema or contact dermatitis. After talking to our friend, I thought that B-15 might do something for her, so I went out and bought her several bottles. The amount of improvement that took place immediately that she began taking the B-15's was so dramatic that it was easily noticed not only by me but by friends who have known her for some time. But the conclusive comment came from her allergy doctor. He asked her what was happening, since she looked so good, and she told him what she was taking. His comment was, 'as far as I know, there is no proven benefit to B-15, but if it helped me the way you are apparently being helped, I would not let anyone dissuade me from taking it.' ''

Yet another grateful testimonial comes from a realtor in Arizona. He writes that ''during one of the periods when I was out of B-15, I was bitten by a Brown Recluse spider in the vicinity of my left ankle. After being treated by a doctor for a period of three months, the swelling of my leg from the knee to the foot was not relieved. At first, I hesitated to take B-15 during the time the doctor directed me to take several other medications, but the swollen leg persisted and finally I decided to take B-15 regardless of the other prescribed medicines. After I'd been taking B-15 for about two weeks, the swelling in my leg subsided and the ulceration caused by the spider bite completely closed and the leg has returned to its natural size.'' (It is interesting, by the way, to note the recurrence of this two-week interval between the time someone begins taking B-15 and the time improvement is noted. It seems to show up in a lot of accounts.)

Of all allergic reactions, asthma can be one of the most terrifying. The victim's chest constricts, each breath becomes an increasingly difficult effort, and he can be reduced to such uncontrollable attacks of wheezing that he feels he is going to suffocate. Yet asthma too seems to respond well to B-15 therapy. Some of the most moving accounts in Dr. Cott's article concern the unhoped-for relief that B-15 has brought to young sufferers from what had been thought hopeless asthmatic conditions. One was a little girl named Ellen, whose mother wrote that she had been diagnosed at two and a half years old as having asthma. She was put on antihistamines, but her attacks got worse, occurring about once every two weeks and lasting two to three days. The doctors tried everything imaginable over the next 18 months—steam tents, antihistamines, even adrenaline. For a while, she did show improvement, but then in the spring of 1965 she began to have such severe attacks that she needed adrenaline quite frequently.

Quite apart from the pain and anxiety of her actual attacks, the condition was impairing Ellen's education and development. Over the next year, she had to be taken out of school nearly half of the time and, when she could go, she always had to be driven to and from the school building because any physical exertion made her breathing even more labored. Needless to say, she could not take gym classes. A sad, confined way indeed for a little child to live.

Then, in January 1971, Ellen started taking B-15. The improvement was almost immediate. By spring, she was showing great advances. She had dispensed with the powerful drugs she had previously needed just to breathe. She was very active riding her bike, swimming, and going on long hikes—all quite unthinkable for her only a few months previously. Thereafter, just as long as she took B-15 regularly, she remained free of asthmatic attacks. The result was a new lease on life. Her mother wrote with gratitude, "We consider this a miracle medication for Ellen."

Yet another enthusiastic testimonial appears in the Food/ Science files. A New Jersey woman wrote happily that "my 12-year-old son, who has had asthma and other allergies since babyhood, told me that he was able to participate in heavy swimming exercises in gym at school without suffering the least symptom for the first time ever—and after taking his first pangamate tablet ever that very morning! Not only that, but after taking his next tablet before bedtime he was able to feel no sense of chest heaviness before falling asleep, something he says never happened before as far back as he can remember!"

A professor of psychology in southern California tells of his reprieve from chronic asthma and bronchial complications. "For over twenty years," he writes, "I have been troubled with periodic asthmatic episodes and have found it increasingly difficult to recover from common colds. Colds always migrated into my chest, resulting in severe bronchitis, asthma, and often bronchial pneumonia. I experienced these cold-bronchitis sequences two or three times each year, and until recently I had not recovered from any of them without medical intervention, usually employing tetracycline and expectorant cough syrups.

"Nor was I getting any better. After several years of treatment at the Kaiser Medical Group Allergy Clinic, and then thorough examination and treatment by a Kaiser pulmonary specialist, I found that by July 1977 I was merely 'getting along' with daily doses of Drixoral and Aminophyllin. Then, through a psychologist friend, I learned of favorable results being obtained in cases of respiratory dysfunction with B-15. Entirely on my own initiative (knowing that my doctor is unsympathetic to such an approach), I ingested my last drugs on July 31, 1977, and on August 1, 1977, I began taking two 50-mg tablets of your B-15 with every meal, along with the supplements that I have been taking regularly for the past four or five years.

"On August 1 and 2, I experienced excruciating headache, and nausea so severe I was forced to remain in bed in a room as darkened as I could manage. The only comparison I can make with the agony I experienced is with the suffering experienced by heroin addicts who drop their habit by going 'cold turkey.' Nevertheless, during those days, I began to experience a freedom in my breathing unlike any I had known for several years, and by August 3, 1977, I felt completely well and was breathing as normally as I could imagine, with a comfort and invigoration that amazed me, a state of being which persists to this date, over a year later.

"At the end of August 1977 I entered a physical fitness program. I recall being unable to run more than one city block without wheezing and becoming exhausted, but by August 13, 1978, I ran a mile in 7′14.88″. I can now very easily run three miles in 27 minutes, with a pulse rate of only 144. I am 53 years old.

"I tried several times in the fall of 1977 to get along on only three B-15 tablets a day, but I experienced bronchial tightness and some wheezing on the reduced dosage. But by February 1978 I was able to get along nicely on three tablets, which is my current daily dosage.

"In August of this year, I returned to the specialist who had examined me before for a follow-up pulmonary examination, which, he informed me, disclosed no change in my condition. He expressed some concern that I had discontinued my medication and warned me that I might expect a migration of head colds into my chest as in the past if I did not avail myself of the support offered by the medication. The fact is that I have had two head colds since August 1, 1977, and in both instances I was fully recovered with no medication whatever—not even aspirin—in less than a week, with all symptoms having been limited to my nasal membranes."

B-15, therefore, just might offer the chance of the breath of life to countless asthma sufferers. But that is far from the end. B-15, in the form of DMG at least, seems to offer help to arthritis victims too. A 71-year-old Ohio man writes: "Four years ago, I was headed for a wheel chair. I had polio when I was nine years old, and it left me with a shrunken right leg. It didn't hamper me too much for the years of my youth, but in time my bad leg began to catch up with me. By 1972, I was beginning to get severe pain in it whenever I did anything strenuous, and soon I began getting pain in it even when I lay down or sat.

"So I went to the doctors. They said arthritis was setting in in that leg, and they gave me some cochicine. I went down to the parking lot and threw it up. Then I found some pills in a local health food store—made from yucca root!—and they did wonders to relieve the pain. When I looked at what was in them, it turned out to be saponin and several vitamins of which B-15 was the most unusual. But I think it was the B-15 that did the trick for me, because subsequently I found your calcium pangamate pills, and started taking them with immediate and spectacular results. All the nerves in my right leg have been regrown—the ones paralyzed when I had polio back in 1918! The itching was infernal while *that* was going on! Muscle regrowth followed. Now, four years later, I have an adolescent right leg, almost as large as the left, and the fifteen-degree layoff of my leg at the knee has been reduced to seven. I have never taken more than one or two calcium pangamate tablets a day, but now I plan to take six a day."

A woman in Tucson adds another striking story. "About half the joints in my fingers were stiff, painful, and enlarged from arthritis," she recounts. "Then I started taking five 50-mg tablets of B-15 a day. Three months later, the swelling had gone down. The stiffness and soreness had first subsided, then disappeared. I reduced my B-15 dose then and in time quit taking it, thinking I no longer needed it. Two months later, I found I had made a mistake. One by one, the finger joints began to swell, becoming painful and stiff again. As soon as I could get more B-15, I started in again on five tablets a day, and in three or four weeks the pain, swelling, and stiffness disappeared once again.

"Again, I reduced my dosage, but this time I stopped at

two tablets a day. I decided that this would be my maintenance dose. I had no trouble with my hands for the next three years, when I ran out of B-15 completely. I've been unable to get more. First a joint in my right, little finger started swelling and hurting, then the index finger on the left hand, followed by the middle and fourth fingers. I have scattered pains that come and go now, including both wrists. I'm afraid this indicates I'll be back in the same or worse condition I suffered four years ago unless my order of B-15 arrives soon. I will never stop taking it as long as it is available to me.''

A Vermont man adds his experience: "In 1965, I had a bad attack of arthritis in my right hand. After taking Vitamin B-15 for about four weeks, the pain was completely relieved, the swellings gone, and my hand was once again normal. In the fall of 1973, I had an arthritis attack in my left knee. This was very severe and I could only walk with the aid of a cane. Once again, I start to take B-15, and within five weeks my knee was back to normal and I am happy to say that the cane remains in the closet.''

It is interesting to note that one of these persons experienced a recurrence of her symptoms whenever she stopped taking B-15, while another was able to discontinue his without trouble when the original arthritis in his hand had cleared. Until controlled experiments are permitted and conducted, we just have to add this datum to the pile of unanswered questions already waiting. Yet the experiences these people relate carry the note of conviction; something very important happened to them, and all indicators seem to point to B-15 as having been intimately involved in their cures. One experiences a rather acute desire to investigate the matter more fully.

One of the most tantalizing reports about B-15 concerns its potential for treating emotionally disturbed and autistic children. Anyone who has ever experienced the tragedy of a severely disturbed child, or who has ever witnessed a friend's pain in seeking to cope with this terrible burden, for which nobody seems to know any cure, will respond feelingly to the hope that B-15 might do something to alleviate this trouble.

And indeed, in the past few years, not only the Soviets but several American doctors have also reported what they believed to be significantly favorable effects from using B-15 in the treatment of retardation, emotional disturbances, and autism in children.

The Soviets, as so often, were the first to look into B-15's possibilities in this area. They took 15 retarded preschool-age children and treated them for one month with 60 milligrams daily of B-15. At the beginning of the treatment, the children were extremely passive and listless, displaying little interest in their surroundings, lacking initiative and showing very underdeveloped speech abilities. At the end of the month, 12 of the 15 children had improved their speech and vocabulary considerably. To assess the extent of other less visible effects, the children were given periodic psychological examinations. These showed that, for most of them, their mental state and intellectual activity had improved. The children became more emotional and active, began to concentrate, got interested in toys and games. The researchers concluded that "pangamate has a pronounced effect on the functional activity of the brain and may find application in the treatment of mentally retarded children."

Intriguing, yes; but 15 children is a pretty small sample, and the evidence the Soviets present is of the sort that might be subject to varying interpretations, since it is, by and large, not subject to quantitative measurement. Still, anything that might help those—victims and parents alike—whose lives are blighted by this tragic condition would seem to be worth a closer look.

And indeed, in this case, the Russians are not the only ones who have found B-15 to hold great promise. Other reports come from closer to home. There's a center in the Midwest—they insist on anonymity—that treats 90 autistic children, some of whom are also retarded. The doctor in charge started administering dimethylglycine to the children, and noticed impressive results. Out of 90 children, 80 responded in significant ways. Some who never could or would speak started slowly to form words. Others who had been totally unaware of their surroundings began reacting to them. Subsequently, the doctor in charge added other nutritional supplements and noticed even greater improvement. One teacher at the center was totally amazed at the children's progress. She thought it was her teaching ability. The doctor says he didn't have the heart to tell her it was the DMG.

Another letter in Da Vinci Laboratories' files is from a California woman, who tells how she began giving B-15 to her three-and-a-half-year-old son at her doctor's suggestion. The boy could not talk. He was still not toilet-trained. But three weeks later, he was using the bathroom unassisted—and he had begun talking. She concluded: "He turned four a little over a month ago, and is acting like a normal four-year-old. He is still slow in his speech, but he is picking up new words every day. I feel that pangamate has been a lifesaver for me."

Among Dr. Allan Cott's case histories are several moving letters from the parents of retarded or emotionally disturbed children. One case is particularly poignant for its account of the severe relapse one child experienced when his supply of B-15 ran out. The child, a four-year-old boy, was originally given B-15 to stimulate speech. He showed an almost immediate positive response. Where before he had been a silent child, with little vocabulary, he now began to form words and to try new ones every day. His mother was delighted, and wrote Dr. Cott of her son's remarkable progress. A month later, she wrote again, a very different letter this time. Her supply of B-15 had run out, and the change in her son after only eight days was drastic. His personality had changed sharply. He seemed severely distressed, lost eye contact, became impatient, and at times destructive. His mother wrote, "It is a terrifying thing to see him go through this. He had come to be a peaceful, happy, easy child. . .but now he looks frightened and runs to us for assurance frequently. I know the B-15 was administered originally to stimulate speech. . .but obviously it has been doing a lot for him that we did not realize fully until this recent relapse." Then she located a new supply of B-15. In twenty-four hours, the boy's crying stopped. In forty-eight hours, his strange behavior disappeared. Thereafter, his speech improved steadily. "It's the most exciting thing I have ever experienced," his mother wrote some months later. "There is no strange look when he tries to talk any more. Instead, he has a big proud smile. Recently, he said something very special for me. 'I love mommy.' "

Dr. Michael Schachter, a Nyack psychiatrist specializing in holistic medicine, also reports good results from using B-15 with brain-damaged children, including those with learning disabilities. He had a very personal reason for getting interested in B-15. "I began working with B-15 because I have a child with cerebral palsy," he says. "My observation has been that B-15 has improved her verbal responses, and parents of my brain-damaged patients tell me too that their children's concentration and verbal production improve with B-15 as part of a comprehensive nutritional program."

Dr. Bernard Rimland, director of the Institute for Child Behavior Research in San Diego, has used B-15 extensively since 1975 in his work with autistic children. In 1976 he wrote to FoodScience/Da Vinci Laboratories telling of the results he had been getting. "I have at this time received reports from the parents of about 15 autistic and autistic-type children on whom Vitamin B-15 has been tried. Frankly I am very impressed, almost amazed, by the very strong and consistent reports I have been receiving describing the effectiveness of the vitamin. Only two or three of the families report no benefits. The others are quite enthusiastic, reporting very significant improvement in many areas, including greater alertness, greater willingness to speak, longer attention span, greater sociability and friendliness to others, as opposed to irritability and withdrawal, which previously characterized the children. Several parents mentioned very significant improvement in the child's sleeping patterns. In a number of instances, the parents had not told teachers, relatives, or neighbors that the child was experimentally taking a new vitamin, and were able to report that these people in the environment had spontaneously commented on the remarkable improvement they had seen in the children."

Dr. Rimland is convinced that B-15 has great possibilities in the treatment of autism. He has a theory that autism may be an allergy of the central nervous system, and thinks that autistic children who respond best to B-15 are those whose basic problem is the consequence of an allergic condition that affects their brain functions. If that is so, then B-15's observed effects in assuaging allergic reactions could also give it immense application in the treatment of autism as well.

Dr. Rimland is already convinced of it. "B-15 gets children speaking better," he says. "They are less irritable and they sleep better. I have gotten such encouraging results from using it in my practice for the past couple of years that I decided to experiment with it on a controlled basis. I asked the parents of some of my patients if they would volunteer their children for such a study. Most of them had been so pleased with B-15's effects when we had been using it as part of an overall program that they were glad to participate. So I've put together a double-blind experiment with about 100 autistic children right now to see if I can gauge B-15's effects on their functioning. Half the children are receiving B-15 and the other half are getting placebos—substances without any medicative content. Neither the children nor their parents know who has received which, but in view of the good results that parents have reported to me just in the general course of treatment, I'm very hopeful that this controlled study will give us some really interesting results to work with."

Finally! A controlled, rigorously designed research experiment! Dr. Rimland's results should be available by the end of 1979. In the meantime, we must rely on the Soviet studies and the grateful testimonials of individuals whose lives seem to have been dramatically changed by B-15. But those alone make one wonder just how much more is waiting to be discovered when the question is at last investigated properly.

The Soviets believe that as valuable as B-15 seems to be in treating a long roster of illnesses, its most important application resides in the treatment of cardiovascular ailments—currently the leading cause of death in the United States. There are more Soviet papers on B-15's uses in treating this group of illnesses than on any other. Indeed, the reports get monotonous after a while; case after case where chest pains are eased, electrocardiograms improved, arterial pressure lowered, and shortness of breath abated. Cases, too, where these symptoms reappeared swiftly after B-15 was withdrawn. Whatever one's objections to the Soviets' style of research, one really has to work at it to remain completely unconvinced of B-15's promise after having read through this bombardment of favorable reports. Maybe the Soviets have exaggerated in places. Maybe other factors helped produce those wonderful results. But it is just about impossible to escape the conviction that *something* is going on there, and something very much worthy of a good close look.

And here again, the Russians are not the only ones contributing reports of good things. Patrick Rings is a New York lawyer in his mid-forties, a partner in a blue-chip Park Avenue firm. "I smoked a bit, drank a bit, worked too hard on occasion for fifteen years," he says. "But I got regular exercise playing squash three times a week and altogether felt fairly fit and energetic until last year. Then I noticed something. Our firm moved into new offices occupying several floors with interior staircases between them. Running up and down those staircases several times a day, I began to get shortness of breath. After a while I quit smoking, but it didn't seem to make any difference. As time went on, those stairs seemed to become tougher to negotiate, and my general overall energy was taking a nose dive. For instance, I couldn't get halfway through a game of squash without having to take a time-out. At first, I thought it was just the aging process, but then I went for a medical checkup and learned that my blood pressure was unusually high and that my cholesterol level was unfavorable. According to the doctor, I simply wasn't getting enough oxygen through my bloodstream. He put me on a low-cholesterol diet, but it didn't seem to make much difference.

"Then, one night about six months ago, I was at a cocktail party one of our clients—a publisher—was giving for the author of a book on nutrition. I got chatting with the author and he mentioned B-15. I figured, what the hell, I'll try it. I started taking it without any expectations whatsoever. At first I didn't notice anything different, but after two or three weeks I realized that I was no longer running out of breath every time I went up the stairs in our office. Also, I was no longer running out of gas at squash. I told my doctor about it but he sort of scoffed, said it was obvious that the new diet that I was on was what was responsible. At first I went along with him, but then I began to wonder. So I got off the diet but stayed on the B-15. Lo and behold, I kept getting better! Today I feel in the pink of health. I had repeat tests last month and my blood pressure was practically back to normal, my cholesterol was down, and my heart signs are all normal. My doctor still believes it was the diet. I'm convinced it was the B-15, and I've been taking it all along. I haven't had the heart to tell him that I've long been off the diet—that I've gone back to smoking, drinking, and eating all the things I'm not supposed to eat, and I still feel great."

Lawyer Rings rejects any suggestion that he might have been the beneficiary of the placebo effect. "Listen, when I started taking B-15, I knew nothing about it. It was just this author of the nutrition book telling me I ought to try it, it might help. I had no idea of what it was supposed to do. I only found out several months later, when my vim and vigor were well on their way back to normal."

Rings' story is by no means an isolated instance. Other even more dramatic cases appear in Da Vinci Laboratories' file of testimonial letters. A woman wrote that her mother had such severe arteriosclerosis that she was unable to walk more than twenty feet without extreme pain in her hips. Also, she was practically unable to do her housework because she could not stand more than five minutes at a time. Then she began taking B-15—600 milligrams a day. "Within four days she was able to walk at least 200 feet without any pain and also was able to do her housework in a nearly normal way. She cut down her intake to 100 mg a day and her condition changed back to the way she had been before taking B-15, only I believe it was even worse now because her right leg became very cold to the touch and felt numb to her. It was quite red, with her toes being almost a blue color.

"We obtained a new supply of B-15 and she immediately began taking 450 mg a day and as before, within about four days, she was again able to walk a 200-foot distance with no discomfort. After about three weeks, we noticed that her right leg was not as red in color or as cold and numb. It is gradually improving. She is feeling much better since taking B-15 and has been able to spend three to four days a week canning vegetables and doing many other things she would never have been able to do without the help of B-15. Words cannot express how very thankful we are."

Dr. Bernard Green tells the story of his patient, Bill, who was 45 and didn't think he would live until 50. "He had a history of heart attacks and high blood pressure," says Dr. Green, "and he had a serious case of arteriosclerosis. I met his doctor at a social gathering, and the man was talking about Bill. He was really worried about him; the man had had four different heart attacks and nothing the doctor had tried seemed to help at all. The doctor had put Bill on Vitamin E and other supplements, in addition to the more standard forms of treatment, but nothing had worked.

"Bill came to see me soon thereafter. He had already quit smoking, and was taking his vitamins regularly. I immediately put him on 20 tablets of B-15 a day, and I also got him into a jogging regimen. I found he was extremely overstressed—which was bad enough—but what was really worse was his inability to cope with the stress. So I got him into biofeedback and meditation, too, to try and minimize some of that stress. Now, with all those things—B-15, jogging, breathing, meditation—I can't swear that any one thing was the governing factor in helping him. But whatever it was, and I personally think the B-15 played a very important part, he has not had an attack since. I saw him about a year later, and he told me his checkups showed he was fine!''

As we shall see later, some controlled experiments now in progress in the United States are at last beginning to substantiate the claims long made for B-15 that it can have significant effects in treating cardiovascular illness. The only pity is that it has taken so long for this sort of evidence to become available. It makes one wonder how much pain, and possibly death as well, might have been avoided if B-15's possibilities had been dispassionately investigated earlier.

The list of diseases goes on. Diabetes is a disease caused by the body's inability to metabolize sugar. The victim loses weight and energy, becomes consumed by thirst, and the body has increasing difficulty healing after injuries. The Soviets reported that *all* diabetics treated with B-15 showed improvement, and that, in light cases, B-15 lowered blood sugar to normal and eliminated it from the urine. The Soviets credited this to B-15's ability to stimulate glucose oxidation. An American doctor in New York City agrees. "It is my opinion," he states, "that calcium pangamate, among its other actions in the body, stimulates glucose oxidation, which accounts for the success the Russians have had with it in the treatment of diabetes. The impairment of an individual's ability to metabolize sugar is the prime contributor to diabetes. Excess sugar becomes a toxin in the system, clogging up the respiration of cells, thickening the bloodstream, and preventing the renal system from doing its normal cleansing work. By increasing blood and cell oxygenation, B-15 effectively counters these pernicious effects and is much more useful than insulin in controlling the disease. I will hazard the prediction that, in time, pangamic acid will make diabetes a disease of the past, like Vitamin C did with scurvy.''

Certainly, the story of one of this doctor's patients suggests that B-15 can have dramatic effects on diabetes. A friend and office colleague of architectural draftswoman Nancy Jackson tells how Nancy was reduced to near somnambulism by the onset of diabetes. "It's amazing about Nancy," she says. "Up until a short time ago, she had become like a zombie around here in the afternoons, and she was not that much more scintillating in the mornings. She walked around slumped over and it took her hours to get anything like a simple rendering done. But within the period of a month, she became a different person, really taking charge of herself and bustling about doing five different jobs at once. Eventually, we found out she was on B-15, and now we're all on it, even the partners in the firm."

Nancy's doctor substantiated the change, pointing out that at the beginning of her treatment, when she started to show improvements in energy and spirits, she was unaware that she was consuming B-15. "Nancy's difficulties came primarily from a pre-diabetic condition that was gradually worsening when I saw her. At first, I put her on a general vitamin therapy program, concentrating on A, the B-Complex, and E, plus the standard diabetes control drugs and strict dietary management. For two or three weeks, she showed no marked improvement except in the sense that her condition stopped worsening. But then I added generous doses of B-15 to the treatment without telling her, and the difference was almost immediate and definitely profound. Her blood sugar level quickly reduced to normal and traces of sugar simultaneously disappeared from her urine samples. This was no placebo influence at work, nor was it spontaneous or coincidental."

Again, a testimonial from the Da Vinci files: A woman in Michigan wrote, "As a diabetic, I started taking Aangamik-15 two months ago. At that time, my sugar count was 278. I recently visited my doctor for my monthly checkup. According to him, my sugar count was normal at 120, and my urine and blood pressure were also normal. My skin tone is better and I walk with greater ease. This is the best my health has been in ten years."

As if this were not enough, reports have also come in that B-15 can help sufferers from emphysema. Listen to another woman writing about her remarkable experience with B-15:

"About nine years ago," she begins, "my doctors confirmed by X-ray and examination that I had emphysema. I was told there was little I could do about it, other than breathing exercises and, later, drugs to dry up excessive fluid. A little discouraging to a woman in her thirties! I had learned about B-15 at a clinic conducted by Mr. Krebs and I decided to take some. I have been taking one a day, almost continually, for a little over a year. The first noticeable improvement was the ability to breathe deeply at full lung capacity. Also, I was able to expectorate all sputum easily."

Then she makes some interesting remarks bearing on the problem of appropriate dosage. "During the first three weeks I started taking it, I felt very tired and wanted to sleep a lot. So, I stopped taking it for about ten days—but again, I started having difficulty breathing. I then started taking only one a day, after breakfast, and this time, besides the ability to clear my lungs and breathe deeply, I had more stamina.

"About a month ago, I decided to stop taking the B-15 to see if it really did make a difference, or if I could get along just as well without it. What a mistake! My breathing became shallow and my sputum was thick and yellow-green. I thought it might be caused by the pollens in the air, so I waited about three weeks, got a lot of rest, didn't overexert myself—and got worse. I started to take the B-15 again, and in about three days I was breathing deeply again. This is proof enough for me, and I personally do not want to stop taking this very beneficial vitamin again."

A young man of 26 in Vermont tells a story of a puzzling malady without a name that threatened to cripple him, but in the end was cured by B-15. "I had an eye problem that nobody seemed to know what it was, let alone how to cure it. I've subsequently come to the conclusion that the problem was that my eye muscles were not getting enough oxygen to function properly, but the effect of that was that I would get so tired from eyestrain that I'd go into dizzy spells. I had to leave graduate school in medicine because I couldn't work through a microscope any more. I would attend two lectures a day and then I'd be in bed for two days. The very last term paper I ever did at the university was done with my eyes closed. I typed the paper while my roommate read me my notes.

"I went to several doctors—Massachusetts General Hospital, several doctors in Canada and Vermont, the Hitchcock Clinic in New Hampshire, about 15 different specialists. I spent in excess of $3,000. They put me in prism therapy, I was wearing trifocals, the whole works. But nothing worked.

"I finally left school and I think I just gave up hope. Then I started taking twelve Aangamik-15 a day, and after a while I realized that my endurance was better. I wasn't getting the severe headaches any more, and I have not yet had a relapse—and that's over a year ago. I don't wear trifocals any more, and I handle a taxing job that requires a lot of reading and record-keeping."

And, finally, there's that subject only slightly behind sex in its ability to command attention: aging. B-15's advocates believe that it can prevent premature aging by inactivating "free radical reactions." What are "free radicals"? Not the Chicago Seven, but certain high-energy fragments of molecules that can damage cellular membranes and other key body components. Some gerontologists believe that they are a major causative factor in the aging process, and the Soviets are deeply impressed by the potential of B-15 in this area. They concluded that it was "a potent stimulant in the control of aging." Dr. Shpirt even stated that he thought in time calcium pangamate would be on the table of every family with people over forty.

Dr. Bernard Green adds some case histories to that effect from his own experience. "This patient, let's call her Joan, was 57 years old. Her husband was in his sixties. He came to me saying she was acting like a child, had very bad arthritis for which she took codeine, was anxious, nervous, had nightmares, needed sleeping tablets to sleep at all, and said she wanted to die. Her diet was the usual American junk one of carbohydrates, sugar, and caffeine. I put her on a diet of fish, eggs, fresh vegetables, fresh fruits, cheese, yogurt, whole wheat grains, with *no* sugar, cakes, pies, salt, or caffeine. Each day, I had her take 300 mg of B-15 (as dimethylglycine) along with brewer's yeast, calcium, B-Complex, and Vitamins E, B-12, and C.

"I saw her twice a week. After a month, she said she felt more alive. After three months, she started to do yoga, including daily asanas [posture exercises], which would have been impossible with her old level of arthritis. Her nightmares disappeared and her depression lifted. Moreover, her sex drive came back, with the result that her marriage revived."

That's a beautiful story, you tell Dr. Green, but how can he be sure that the B-15 was so important when he had changed her diet in so many other ways?

"Good point," he replies, "but the reason I think so is that I've had other patients in which the B-15 was *added* to a pre-existing regime that had not brought results, and adding the B-15 did. Let's call this patient Sheila. She was 67 years old, a widow, and for six months out of the year she was chronically depressed. She lay in bed having to be fed intravenously, her memory was failing to the point where she couldn't remember what she had eaten at breakfast. She also had grandiose fantasies about being a great leader. When spring arrived, she would come out of her cocoon enough to walk around the house, but she never left it, and she still said she wanted to die.

"Now, when she came to me, she was *already* on a vitamin regimen, but it had produced no results. When I added ten B-15's a day, however, the results began to show very dramatically. She now has a 71-year-old boy friend, and they're going on a Caribbean cruise together. She recently asked me whether I thought they should get married or just live together!"

Well, where does all this leave us? In a word, wondering. Nobody will maintain that the evidence described in this chapter is conclusive. It consists instead of a wide assortment of clinical observations and personal testimonials, plus the results of the Soviet studies.

The scattered clinical evidence reported by American medical practitioners is frequently arresting and provocative, but it *is* scattered, resulting from the observations and conclusions of numerous individuals working under different conditions. Moreover, it almost always describes results obtained by using B-15 in combination with other substances. This is chiefly due to the fact that at present in the United States those members of the medical community who are the most enthusiastic about B-15 represent a new breed of doctor—specialists in what is known as "holistic" medicine. Holistic physicians subscribe to a medical philosophy that views a specific degenerative organic disease as being the result of immunological and metabolic imbalances in the *whole* system (thus the term holistic) of the victim. A cancer, for example, is seen not so much as the emergence of the malignant cells forming the tumor as it is the manifestation of one or more systemic short circuits unleashed by a general assault on the entire immunogenic and metabolic network. Specific orthodox therapies can be useful, but alone they have a high degree of failure—one that has already been documented. This is because, in holistic terms, treating the specific cancer site is not enough. The victim's whole system must be treated in order to reverse the process that allowed the cancer to take root. To the holistic physician, no component part of the body can be considered medically except in the context of the whole body. Accordingly, "whole-body" therapy is the course to follow in the treatment of any disease.

Holistic medicine places maximum value on nutritional and environmental revisions in the patient to restore immunogenic and metabolic balances. Only when these balances are restored will true healing occur, as opposed simply to the alleviation of symptoms. All other methods of healing—surgery, pharmaceutical therapy, and the like—are simply of the stopgap variety. The entire human system is organized and structured through its immunogenic and metabolic networks to fend off the usual bacterial, viral, and other attacks on it that can cause disease. But these networks have not evolved fast enough to neutralize the carcinogens and other disease-producing substances imposed on them by the rapidly changing quality of our national diet and environment. Which is why serious degenerative disease is on the increase rather than diminishing.

This approach to medicine implies that the holistic physician is going to use a wide variety of methods and substances in his treatment of any particular disease. In this multidirectional approach, B-15 becomes one of a battery of therapeutic tools designed to rectify the entire body system, rather than a specific administered in response to an identified cluster of symptoms. That means that the holistic physician's results are not going to produce solid statistics as to the benefits of B-15 when used alone. And because each holistic physician is likely to use his own combination of therapeutic substances and methods, his results may not be comparable with those of other physicians who may have used a different combination. Therefore, we don't come out with an answer to the synergism question either—for even if one grants that B-15 does work better in combination with other things, it has not been clearly established *which* things these might be. All one can say with certainty, then, is that when combined with dozens of other natural substances, including vitamins, minerals, and certain foods, and used in conjunction with certain quasi-medical system-cleansing techniques such as enemas, liver rinses, and mind relaxation, B-15 has become a significant ingredient in holistic therapy.

Just the same, the possibilities *are* tantalizing; and anybody truly interested in the easing of pain and the curing of disease must find himself curious to define the true boundaries of B-15's potential. It is all but impossible moreover, to resist the impact of all those intensely personal testimonials about how B-15 has changed lives and relieved illnesses of the most diverse nature. They too may be called unscientific and subjective—but does that justify our dismissing them entirely? *Something* seems to be going on there. It certainly seems worth the gamble to find out just what it really is.

One last story may sum up the matter. It's Greg Hausner speaking, the president of a book-wholesaling company, a high-powered, high-energy dynamo who always seemed able to feed off the pressures of his competitive business. A year or so ago, he suddenly found himself in an acute physiological decline. "I'd gone down to Acapulco for a week's vacation after the Christmas season with my wife. When I arrived, I was my usual charged-up self, feeling terrific because the season had been so great and looking forward to a little tennis, a little sailing, a little golf, and so on. When I go on vacation, I stay active and just leave the cares of the office behind. Well, about midway through my stay, I caught the Mexican bug—you know, that gastrointestinal thing they call Montezuma's revenge. It completely wiped me out and I had to spend three extra days there, in bed, before I could make my way back to the States.

"Once I was back, I couldn't seem to shake the thing. The diarrhea and stomach cramps had disappeared and all my systems seemed to be normal, but I never got my energy back. Jesus, I dragged myself through January and February hardly able to get anything accomplished. I'd wake up in the morning feeling half-dead, I'd schlep into the office late and not really caring what was going on, I'd fall asleep at my desk before lunch, I'd be a wreck by three in the afternoon, and on the train ride back to my suburban home, I'd often fall asleep and end up missing my stop. One time there I even slept all the way to the end of the line.

"Then, in March, I took a business trip to California. I had one drink on the plane and passed out. The pilot landed in Chicago so I could be taken off and put in a hospital. Stayed in the hospital for two days, in the coronary ward, scared shitless, but they couldn't find a damned thing wrong with me. So after two days, feeling better but still completely washed out, I got on another plane and continued my trip. I got talking to the stewardess about what happened and it was she who told me about B-15. She said all the stewardesses and flight crews were taking it because it helped them overcome the effects of high-altitude pressurized cabins and jet lag, things like that. She thought I might just have been suffering from 'flight fever.'

"She gave me a handful of pills and I took them and I got to California in one piece but still as sluggish as ever. Then, when it came time for me to fly back, I remembered what she said and bought a bottle of pills. I kept stuffing them into myself on the flight back to New York, and when I got off the plane at Kennedy I thought I felt a little better. That lasted for a day or so, and then I began to feel worse again. I finally checked with a doctor and he could still find nothing wrong, just said something about male menopause, gave me a shot of gamma globulin, and put me on some B vitamins. I went along like that for a few weeks and felt a little more lively but not much, nothing like my old self. Then one day, as I was taking some of the doctor's vitamins, I noticed the bottle of B-15 pills in the corner of my medicine cabinet. I figured since I was taking other B vitamins, I might as well throw down a few of the B-15's as well. I did that every day for a couple of weeks, more to get rid of the B-15's than anything else, and it wasn't but a few days before I began to feel *really* better. No more dizzy spells, no more heart palpitations, no more dragging my ass around and falling asleep in the middle of the day.

"At first, I attributed it to the doc's regular vitamin therapy finally taking hold. But after I ran out of the B-15's, I began to slide back. That's when I thought there might be a connection. So I got more B-15's and the same thing happened—I started to feel infinitely better again. When my doctor's vitamins petered out, I kept up on the B-15's and I've been getting better and better ever since. The upshot is that I've put some money into a company that makes calcium pangamate and I'm running around the country half the time promoting the stuff. Don't ask me how it works or why. Just believe me when I say it works. At least, it worked on me, and now I know dozens of other people who are taking it on my urging and who find it works for them too."

And that's just the point: a lot of people have found that B-15 *works*. Do we call them liars? Do we say they are deluded? Or do we take a closer look and see just what it is that is happening? For the pragmatic nation we pride ourselves on being, the answer seems to be obvious. We didn't get to be the world's foremost scientific power by ignoring controversial scientific questions. Maybe it's time we really bit into this one.

6

B-15
and Cancer

If there's one thing that raises emotions to the boiling point in the B-15 debate, it's the assertion by some of B-15's supporters that it can help in the treatment of the most dread disease of all: cancer. A bold claim indeed. But it has a basis in respectable scientific theory. Remember Dr. Felix Warburg's theory that cancerous cells are cells that have adapted to oxygen starvation by learning to survive on glucose rather than oxygen? If that is so, then B-15 might very possibly help to prevent cancer, because by increasing the available oxygen in the body system, it would make the switch to glucose that much less necessary.

As violently controversial as this idea may be now—and it arouses some pretty strong emotions—a few years ago it would have been just about unthinkable. The official medical view of cancer's origin has undergone some dramatic changes in recent years. Where decades of earlier research have gone into exploring the theory that cancer is caused by a virus or some other sort of invasion of the body by outside agents, the view is gaining ever wider acceptance in the medical community that most cancers find their source in cell anomalies brought about by faulty cell nutrition. Its incidence is increasing not because some mysterious virus has become more prevalent but because with the onward march of industrialization in this century, we have come to consume ever more highly processed, low-bulk, heavily sugared foods, and to breathe ever more polluted air. All this combines to alter normal cell metabolism, spawning cancerous cells which then attack healthy cells and, through a process of chemical proselytization, turn them into cancerous cells.

This new view of cancer, indeed, has been publicly endorsed by some of the most authoritative figures in cancer research. In June 1978, Dr. Arthur Upton, director of the National Cancer Institute, testified in Washington before a Senate subcommittee looking into the state of federally funded cancer research today, asking why, after so many tens of millions of dollars had been spent, so little progress had been made in the "war on cancer." It was Upton who declared that "there is definitely a direct link between the great majority of cancer cases in this country and diet." It might be a better idea, he told the inquiring senators, for the government to direct most of its research funding at developing a preventative rather than seeking the ever-elusive cure. Dr. Upton's statement was corroborated by his fellow-witness, Dr. Donald Frederickson, the director of the National Institutes of Health, who stated that roughly two thirds to three quarters of all cancer cases in America are directly related to our eating and drinking habits.

Revise diet and improve air quality, these two pillars of the American medical establishment were saying, and the current cancer epidemic will wane. A revolutionary admission indeed. American medicine has traditionally been notorious for its rejection of nutritional and dietary considerations as factors in the genesis and treatment of disease, whereas these have retained at times quite honorable positions in the medicine of other countries. We have instead prided ourselves—at times quite justly—on the triumphs of our medical machines, our surgical techniques, our arsenal of seemingly miraculous drugs. These have grown out of our general insistence in the past that sickness came from *outside* the body and that therefore the way to treat it was by introducing counteracting factors, also from the outside. The notion that sickness might frequently be a creation of the body itself has run at such cross-purposes to this outlook that it has often met the most heated rejection.

But here are two prominent representatives of established medicine saying precisely that—and in a very public forum to boot. The effect of their statements is to refocus our attention on changing our life style in our increasingly industrialized world, on reconsidering the way we eat, and on improving the air we breathe.

But that is easier said than done. Our present diet and air quality are the results of almost two hundred years of intensive industrial and technological development. They represent economic interests totaling billions of dollars. To revise them in any thoroughgoing way would require an impossibly expensive turnabout of the nation's industrial base. In short, we are more or less stuck with them, whatever improvements in detail we might manage.

Then, ask some of B-15's advocates, wouldn't the next best thing be to discover a preventative? If one can't eliminate cancer-causing toxins, perhaps one could at least find ways of neutralizing or counteracting them? And might not B-15— with its oxygenating abilities—be a way of doing that? There were those who tried to get that question brought up at the Senate subcommittee hearings. Lobbyists for the vitamin industry tried hard to get several senators to ask Drs. Upton and Frederickson why little or no research had been conducted into B-15 as a possible cancer preventative. The politically wary senators declined to pose the question. But a subcommittee staffer later asked Upton about it off the record. Upton laughed wryly and answered, "That's all we need—to start fooling around with quack medicines at this stage of the game."

A striking reaction, to say the least. Just why should this supposedly serious-minded scientist conclude that B-15 was a "quack medicine," when no serious effort has been made in this country to find out *what* it is? Is not the proper scientific attitude to inquire first and judge afterwards? Why then this strong, a priori prejudice against B-15, a prejudice strong enough to prevent even research that might *disprove* the claims made for B-15 once and for all?

A lot of the difficulty is guilt by association. Ernest Krebs, who claims to have discovered B-15, was also the discoverer of a substance even more violently controversial: Laetrile. Not only that, he reported having found both substances in the same place: the kernels of apricot pits. From the beginning, Krebs claimed that Laetrile acted in the body similarly to pangamic acid, and that by restoring oxygen to cancer-diseased cells, it enabled the cells to revert to normal respiration. But what made Laetrile particularly antagonistic to cancer, Krebs contended later, was the very cyanide contained in it that led the FDA to ban the substance. According to Krebs, Laetrile is a highly selective substance that attacks only cancerous cells. When it is ingested and then absorbed by normal cells, an enzyme called rhodanase detoxifies the cyanide, which is eventually excreted in the urine. But cancer cells are completely lacking in rhodanase and are instead surrounded by another enzyme, beta-glucodase. This enzyme releases the cyanide from the Laetrile at the site of the malignancy. Therefore, said Krebs, Laetrile attacks only cancerous cells.

Krebs further theorized that Laetrile would be particularly effective in curing lymphatic cancer, or Hodgkin's disease, because of the way it is stored and absorbed by the body. Oral doses of Laetrile are thought not to be affected by acid-digestive action of the stomach but are believed to pass directly into the intestine, where they are acted upon by bacterial enzymes. The enzymes in the intestine decompose the substance into four components, two of which are sugar and one cyanide. These components are absorbed directly into the lymphatic system and then circulated through the rest of the body. Because the cyanide's entryway is the lymphatic system, the lymph glands—the site of Hodgkin's disease—are the first organs to receive its allegedly cancer-destroying benefits.

The FDA has always borne down hard on the question of Laetrile's potentially toxic effect. When it banned Laetrile and made it illegal for doctors to administer it, it used the possibly harmful effects of cyanide build-up as its justification, claiming that research had failed to show that the substance was *not* dangerous. This, however, was less than straightforward, because there *is* research evidence attesting to Laetrile's non-toxicity. Dr. Dean Burke, then chief cytologist of the National Cancer Institute, tested Laetrile's toxic effects and stated that it "is remarkably non-toxic . . . compared with virtually all cancer chemotherapeutic agents currently in use."[1] For that matter, if possible toxicity were all there were to it, one would have to ban a lot of other cancer-treatment agents around, as anyone can attest who has witnessed the side-effects of chemotherapy.

Yet one can understand some of the practising physician's reluctance to use the unproven substance Laetrile when other established therapies do exist, some of which *are* known to cure. The price of delay or error in treating cancer is, of course, death—not to mention a malpractice suit! Yet the pain associated with some of these therapies can make one pause, too, and wonder if there might not be some better way. Since no conclusive research has been allowed into Laetrile's curative abilities, somebody seeking an alternative to radiation or chemotherapy is confronted by agonizing uncertainties: on the one hand, there *are* reports of Laetrile's having helped cancer sufferers, sometimes dramatically; on the other hand, nobody can point to any scientific evidence to confirm those reports. So the search for alternate therapies can generate some tragic situations. A highly publicized instance of this was the so-called "Hofbauer case."

In the fall and winter of 1977, the city of Albany, New York, was caught up in the medical drama of eight-year-old Joseph Hofbauer—"Little Joey" as the local newspapers and television commentators quickly dubbed him. Joey Hofbauer had recently contracted the form of cancer known as Hodgkin's disease, a malignancy of the lymphatic glands.

---

[1] "Laetrile—An Answer to Cancer?" *Prevention* Magazine, December 1971.

Within the previous fifteen years, medical science had developed techniques of treating Hodgkin's disease, using a combination of chemotherapy and radiation, that by 1977 rendered this once surely fatal ailment curable, or controllable, in a great majority of cases. This was particularly true in the so-called Stage 1 phase of the disease, when the cancerous tumors are still confined to the lymphatic glands and have not metastasized, or spread, into other parts of the body.

When Joey Hofbauer's cancer was first diagnosed by physicians at the Albany Medical Center, his doctors determined that he was still in Stage 1 and stood a great chance of being cured through the standard series of chemotherapy and radiation treatments, which are known in the medical world as "conventional therapy." They consulted with the lad's parents and recommended that he be immediately started on conventional therapy. John Hofbauer, his father, balked. He had heard about the effects of chemotherapy and radiation—constant headaches, continual nausea and vomiting, hair loss, hallucinations, and the like—and decided that it would be inhumane to submit his barely comprehending eight-year-old son to such agonies. The doctors were astonished. What could be more inhumane, they asked, than to withhold the boy from a proven treatment for the sake of sparing him some temporary discomfort? Without the treatment, chances were horribly overwhelming that Joey would die once the cancer began to spread, as it inevitably would.

John Hofbauer remained adamant in his disagreement with Joey's physicians. He would not submit him to conventional therapy. Instead, he would seek a cure through Laetrile and "nutritional therapy." He had heard and read about the great successes certain foreign medical jurisdictions had recently reported with Laetrile in the treatment and cure of cancer. "You're crazy," said one of Joey's doctors, reminding the senior Hofbauer that Laetrile had long before been adjudged useless in the battle against cancer. "You're not only crazy," added the doctor, "but if you deprive this boy of a genuine chance to be saved, you are criminally insane."

"Sorry," replied John Hofbauer, "but he's my son and I intend to do what I think is best for him."

"But he'll die!" shouted the doctor.

An arguable claim, Hofbauer shot back. But better that Joey should die without pain than live with pain. Whereupon Hofbauer, a man of modest means, withdrew his life savings and flew off with his son to the island of Jamaica to seek Laetrile treatment.

John Hofbauer was well aware of the long history of governmental hostility to Laetrile. It was this very history that fostered Laetrile's appeal to him with respect to the treatment of his son's cancer. Hofbauer, a God-fearing, rock-ribbed conservative, had grown increasingly bitter during his adult years at what he viewed as the expanding and insidious intrusion of governmental regulation and control in the life of the average citizen. When he scorned Joey's doctors' urgings that the boy receive immediate conventional therapy, he was not only acting out of his unique sense of concern for his son but was also making a political statement—one tinged with religious overtones. "There is a higher authority in my life than the government," he was saying in effect. That authority was God. God was the dictator of Hofbauer's conscience, and his conscience told him that he could not submit his son to the pain of chemotherapy and radiation treatments. If his son died as a consequence, then that was God's wish. In the meantime, he would do everything he could, within the bounds of his conscience, to save Joey. The government had no right to intrude in the matter.

While Hofbauer was in Jamaica with Joey at a clinic there, the boy was fed daily doses of Laetrile and other nutritional supplements; meanwhile, the doctors in Albany complained of the father's decision to members of the New York State Department of Health and the Social Services Department. When Hofbauer returned home with his son ten days later, he found himself more embroiled with the government than he could ever have imagined. The state had instituted a suit against him in a local family court charging him with child abuse and petitioning the court for custody of Joey so that it could, through its Social Services Department, put him into conventional therapy. Hofbauer vigorously contested the action. There ensued weeks of bitter legal battle, in and out of court, as "little Joey"—now the subject of intense press attention—was first wrenched from the arms of his father by court decree and temporarily delivered over to the custody of the state, and then temporarily returned to his family by a countermanding order. After several evidentiary hearings, during which violently conflicting "expert" testimony was taken from a number of medical practitioners on the vices and virtues of Laetrile, and the question of the privilege of a provably responsible parent to determine the rights and welfare of his child as against the state's constitutional responsibility to guarantee such rights and welfare was debated, the inevitable compromise was struck by the presiding judge. He allowed Joey to continue exclusively on Laetrile treatment, but ordered that his condition be monitored weekly by conventional doctors representing the court and the state. The court reserved the right, at the first sign of a worsening of Joey's condition, to order him into conventional therapy.

"The stupidest and most criminal decision possible!" cried one doctor to the press. "It's the kiss of death. By the time there's a sign of worsening, it will most likely be too late for chemotherapy." The sentiment was echoed by countless other conventional practitioners, as well as by lawyers for the state who busied themselves with higher-court appeals.

In the meantime, Joey Hofbauer was delivered by his father into the care of Dr. Michael Schachter, a psychiatrist practicing in downstate Nyack. Schachter (who has been already mentioned in Chapter 5 in connection with his work dealing with brain-damaged children) started Joey on a regimen of Laetrile and other vitamin-nutritional supplements. During the months that followed, the state continued to seek custody of Joey, claiming that his condition was demonstrably deteriorating, while John Hofbauer continued to resist, insisting that his son was actually getting better. In early 1978,

Hofbauer, threatened again by the prospect of losing custody of Joey, moved his family from New York State and thus, presumably, from the jurisdiction of its courts. Most of the doctors who examined Joey prior to his removal from New York's jurisdiction contended that his cancerous lymph glands had indeed become worse during the Laetrile treatment administered by Dr. Schachter, that his condition had progressed to the Stage 2 phase, and that he was doomed to die if continued solely on Laetrile therapy. Dr. Schachter, on the other hand, insists that even though Joey's condition did not markedly improve, it became stabilized under his treatment and that further Laetrile therapy would likely bring about remission.

Dr. Hugh Leahy, a retired Albany pediatrician, commenting on the Hofbauer case, speaks eloquently for those who believe Laetrile is a dangerous delusion. "I have treated children for close to fifty years as a practising physician," he says, "and not a year went by in all that time when I didn't encounter a seriously sick child—sometimes two or three cases a year—whose parents balked at the recommended proven treatment and decided to take matters into their own hands. In those days, we doctors did not go to the state to try to protect the child, since the state, except in unusual cases such as clearly insane parents, would not back us up. So we had to swallow our tongues and our anger and watch these children die. As far as I'm concerned, these parents were guilty of murder, and I'm glad to see the state step in as it did in the Hofbauer case. I only despair that the state failed to win its action and thereby lost access to the boy. I don't care what the constitutional issues are. As far as I'm concerned, a parent definitely does not have the right to play God with his or her child's life. And I don't care what the motivations are—whether they're political, religious, or just plain downright anti-doctor.

"We obviously can't legislate everything that parents do to their children. We can agree, for example, that teaching children to hate mindlessly is terrible, but it is something that is beyond society's ability to realistically control through law.

But at the same time, parents cannot be free to do whatever they want to do with their children. If a father throws his five-year-old son into a pool thinking that this is the only way he'll learn to swim, and he says 'sink or swim,' and the boy drowns, the father is liable. The father might say, 'Well, I thought the boy would come up after he'd been down at the bottom for two or three minutes.' But that would not get him off the hook. If it could be proved that the boy did not know how to swim, and that the father threw him into the water, and that he made no effort to rescue him after he was on the bottom for more than a few moments, that father is guilty of manslaughter at least under the law.

"Now, I'm not going to make any such characterization about Joey Hofbauer's parents in this case. But I will say that, based on my long experience, any parent who jeopardizes his or her ill but statistically curable child's life by withholding that child from legitimate and proven treatment is in the same boat. Under even the strictest constitutional interpretation of the law, the parent should be required to submit the child to treatment or deserves to relinquish custody to someone or some organization that will. People who claim to act out of religious reasons and who say that God is the ultimate authority in the fate of their children conveniently forget that it is the very same God that put gifted doctors on this earth to save lives.''

But, then, one asks: Dr. Leahy, what about Laetrile? Isn't it possible that it might cure Joey? "Listen, I've seen every new drug, curative and palliative, that's come down the line in the last fifty years. A few fulfilled their promise, but most of them turned out to be duds. Give me documented proof that shows that Laetrile has cured a case of cancer. Until you can, I'll stick to proven therapies that at least have a chance, whether they be surgical or non-surgical. Let me put it to you this way. Suppose your child was diagnosed as having cancer—say Hodgkin's. Or suppose you were. What would you do? Would you submit yourself or your child to the proven therapies? The ones that you know will at least give you a chance of survival? Or would you say, 'Well, they may cause me some discomfort, so I'll skip them and go for Laetrile treatment, even though Laetrile has not been shown to have cured a single case of cancer.' Tell me you'd opt for the Laetrile.''

It's pretty hard to say yes—but one can still feel revulsion at the agonies of chemotherapy, too. What about prevention? Was it possible that Laetrile might act in such a way as to prevent cancer?

"Wouldn't that be glorious," says Dr. Leahy. "God, if I thought that was even remotely possible, I'd have been taking B-17, as it's sometimes called, for years. But enough time has passed for its promoters to have documented their claim that it prevents cancer, or certain kinds of cancer. As far as I know, there has been no documentation. So I can only say that Laetrile is about as effective in preventing cancer as orange juice or chocolate candy.''

There we are again. There's no scientific proof; therefore, Laetrile must be worthless. In instituting its original ban on Laetrile, the FDA declared that no disinterested study had been conducted proving that Laetrile had ever cured a single case of cancer, let alone prevented one. And the result of the FDA's ban, which went into effect in the late 1960's, has been that there has *still* been no such research conducted in any American medical circles—establishment or maverick—that would either prove *or* discredit the claims made for Laetrile, although reports do come in from overseas of such results. The FDA congratulates itself on having successfully forestalled what one of its administrators called "the development of a national hysteria over a false miracle cure for cancer. Had we sanctioned the stuff, tens of thousands more cancer victims would be dead of the disease today instead of having been rehabilitated through medically valid treatments.'' Yet there's an element of circularity in all this. Laetrile (like B-15) is declared "medically invalid" because no research has ever proven its claims—yet such research was banned before any of the claims could be properly investigated. One begins to think of Catch-22.

Right about here, we stumble on an odd aspect of the Laetrile controversy. It turns out that back in the early 1960's the FDA *did* grant permission to Biozymes International, Ltd. to conduct research into Laetrile's effects on humans—and then, a couple of weeks later, revoked that permission without explanation. Dom Orlandi tells the story this way: "They gave us an IND number. That means Investigational New Drug, and it means you can use the substance on humans. They wanted us to test it, giving some patients Laetrile and others not. To me, that seems pretty cruel, to tell somebody you're giving them Laetrile and then not give it to them, but anyway that's the way they wanted us to do it. Then this guy comes to us, one of the experimental subjects, and he offers us $25,000 on top of the treatment costs if we will guarantee to him that he'll be one of the people to be given Laetrile during the course of the experiment. We told him we couldn't do it, of course. Just after that, our IND number got pulled. I don't know why, but my guess is that that guy had a friend that was the Surgeon General or something. So I think they just got together and got the FDA to pull our number." Orlandi's suspicions may be right, or they may be wrong, but one cannot help being intrigued by the fact that the FDA did at one time approve research that it now so adamantly opposes.

Certainly, there are some straws in the wind that suggest there's something there worth investigating. For example, there's Dom Orlandi saying, "My mother's doctors told us she had to have a double radical mastectomy because the lumps in her breasts might turn malignant. Well, my mother has two breasts today and they're both healthy, thanks to Laetrile. Furthermore, where she had previously had a long history of non-malignant tumors, she doesn't have those any more either." There are also all the reports that have trickled in over a period of years of how Laetrile has helped cancer sufferers throughout the country—to the point where some members of the medical community are finally beginning to suggest that it might be used with terminal cancer patients for whom all other remedies have proved ineffective. Yet, so far, where *both* Laetrile and B-15 are concerned, the government and the biomedical community seem to display the same resistance towards even asking the question, let alone debating the answer.

Why the allergy to inquiry? A West Virginia doctor believes it's a matter of sheer economic self-interest. "They always point to the Sloan-Kettering research findings that Laetrile is useless in treating cancer," he notes impatiently. "Well, any serious scientific researcher can poke holes by the dozen through that report. It just simply does not prove the case. Let's face it, cancer is big business these days. It's a very profitable part of the biomedical industry. I seriously question if they *want* to cure it."

How about researching B-15 then? There are doctors who consider the United States government's resolute refusal to explore B-15's potential a national tragedy. "Gross negligence on the part of the government," says one, a medical nutritionist and biochemist. "Given the findings of the Russians in 1965 on diabetes and cardiovascular problems and their responsiveness to calcium pangamate, the government should have leaped onto the possibilities of B-15 in cancer research. Just recently, the National Institutes of Health and the National Cancer Institute have come out with the assertion that almost three quarters of all the cancer that occurs is caused by nutritional and environmental factors. Even now it's not too late to get into some hard-nosed studies on B-15. Take ten thousand people—a cross-section of the population. Have half of them take B-15 for the next ten years and have the other half go without it. At the end of that time, compute the number of B-15 users who have contracted cancer and measure that figure against the number of non-users who got cancer. Then compare the figures with a random equivalent segment of the overall population. If after ten years, the 5,000 B-15 users showed only a slight decrease in cancer contraction as compared with a random sample of 5,000 non-users, it would be highly significant. We would know we were onto something. But the goddamn government has closed its eyes to this thing, and such studies are far too expensive for private-sector support."

Contends another physician, "Cancer is much too complex and variegated a disease for anyone to expect to find a preventive or even a cure in a single substance. But I have seen from my own practice that the administration of B-15 in certain patients has had remarkable effects in the quelling of certain chronic illnesses. I have had patients who would come to me once every month or so for years with outbursts of chronic ulcers, or bronchial problems, or gastrointestinal ailments. In many of these cases, B-15 has put an end to the recurring nature of these illnesses, and I see these patients much more seldom now, and usually for something else. This is proof to me that pangamic acid is a valuable medical substance. Whether it can prevent cancer or not, or certain kinds of cancers, is a question that remains to be scientifically determined. I can say, however, that since I've been prescribing B-15 to my large bloc of patients, I have been diagnosing fewer and fewer cancers among them. This is over the last five years. Whether it has anything to do with B-15 or not also remains to be scientifically determined. Although I don't have the resources to prove it, I have reported on it in the hope that someone or some organization with more financial clout will take up the matter and investigate it."

There again is the tantalizing suggestion that B-15 can do something remarkable, but also an absence of hard scientific proof one way or the other. How about the drug companies, then? Wouldn't one expect them to latch on to something that seemed to promise as much as some think B-15 does? Apparently they don't think it's a live prospect, although none of them specifies which chemical formulation it was that they tested. Unless it was N,N-Dimethylglycine (the FoodScience formula), the chances are strong that what they looked at was the synthetic analog, DIPA, and if so, this might possibly help cast some light on the effects to be expected from the two main contenders for the title of "the Real B-15." But the company representatives don't distinguish between these two formulations in voicing their disdain. And disdain it is. Take the articulate representative of the pharmaceutical industry, a high-level officer of Pfizer, who for professional reasons wishes to remain anonymous. Let's call him Mr. Pfizer.

"It's true," he says, "we looked into B-15 a long time ago when word first began to circulate in the scientific community about its alleged curative and preventative properties. To a certain extent, all of the pharmaceutical companies, at least in their marketing operations, are in the business of selling illusions. Much of our profits derive from the general public's obsession with feeling better, looking better, and so on. B-15 would have been a natural for us, even if it only did a tenth of what was originally claimed for it. We would have paid a small fortune for the right to manufacture and sell it, no question about it. So we ran some extensive secret tests on it in our labs, and we learned that it was absolutely worthless. I can say, without fear of scientific contradiction, that B-15 generates absolutely no chemical action within the body other than the ordinary ones. By that I mean it goes through your system just like everything else you eat and eventually gets disposed of by your waste organs, without having one smidgen of beneficial effect on your cells or tissues. All this business about increased oxygen-uptake and the diminution of sugar metabolism is the product of someone's fertile imagination. If we had found that B-15 had any worth whatsoever in cure, prevention, or just making someone feel better, we could easily have gotten the FDA to change its position on it and made it a marketable substance. But as far as we were concerned, the FDA was right. It's absolutely worthless. We may sometimes pander to the public's illusions, and we may even once in a while create illusions to capture the public's interest in something we market that has *some* value. But we are not out to lie to the public. We are not out to make profits by selling the public something that is completely valueless."

Interviews with officials of several other large pharmaceutical companies elicited similar statements of disdain for B-15 as a therapeutic chemical agent. As a marketing vice-president of the Hoffman-LaRoche Company remarked, echoing the sentiments of Mr. Pfizer, "We looked into B-15 thoroughly years ago and found that it was totally without effects of any kind. Sure, considering the public's fascination with it today, we could put out a compound, call it 'B-15' or 'pangamic acid,' and probably make a lot of money. We could combine it with calcium or niacin or any number of other substances that would give the user a definite feeling that something was happening in his body as a result of taking it. But the effect would be purely from the chemicals or minerals it was combined with. We could put some benzedrine-like substance into it, for instance, and when you swallowed, you'd say, 'Hey, this stuff really works!' But we'd also be defrauding you. Our scientists determined conclusively through lab experiments that pangamic acid, whether alone or in combination with other natural chemicals, has no unusual chemical effect upon the tissues and organs of the human body. What you get from pangamic acid is no different than what you get from eating an apricot. No doubt, eating an apricot can be good for you—it gives you a lot of desirable nutritional elements. But so does eating an apple or a peach.''

Says Derrik van Nimwegen, a former marketing bigwig with Bristol-Myers, the giant manufacturer of popular over-the-counter medications, ''There was some interest in the stuff when I was with Bristol back in the early 1970's, but lab studies by our scientists quickly put it to rest. It all had to do with its molecular properties, and it was found that pangamate produced no unusual molecular phenomena in any kind of animal tissues. Nor did any unusual kinds of molecular events occur when it was combined in test tubes with other substances. Having learned about B-15 from the inside, so to speak, I have watched with some amusement the tidal wave of interest in it in recent years. As far as I can determine, it's all a matter of self-fulfilling prophecy. Now that nutrition, diet, and environment have become the bugaboos in disease epidemiology—and I don't doubt for a minute that they should be—people are wildly casting about for magic nutritional antidotes. That people's consciousness has been raised about these things is good. But the bad thing is that they tend to latch on to anything that the nutritional propagandists claim holds the answer. The nutritional lobby, as I would call it, has gotten a message across about B-15 that flies in the face of scientific evidence. Scientists are for the most part a quiet, reticent group, and they're not going to mobilize to inform the public that everything that's being claimed for B-15 is a lot of scientific rot. They've seen so many other miracle cures come down the pike and fizzle out that they couldn't care less. They figure the fad for B-15 will run its course, just like everything else has. But the uninformed public at large—well, what do they know? They're ready and willing to believe anything. If someone with some apparent authority says that something is good for you, they'll believe it and they'll begin taking it. And maybe they'll even feel better. But usually that's because they have been propagandized into believing that they're supposed to feel better. When someone believes that he is supposed to feel better as a result of taking something, in nine cases out of ten he *will* feel better. Some of the young marketing hotshots at Bristol recommended that the company put out a version of B-15 and accompany it with a big advertising campaign. But wiser heads in the executive suite prevailed, reasoning that the product would eventually be proven worthless and that the company would end up with egg on its face."

Crushing testimony indeed, it would seem. Yet an outstanding Baltimore cardiovascular surgeon who has worked with B-15 and considers it of great promise offers a strikingly different perspective. "Why have the pharmacological companies not followed up on B-15?" he asks. "Well, for one thing, it's *very* expensive—it takes about five million dollars to develop a new drug. Then, because of the FDA problem, you could be sued. And you might discover in the course of your research that it is one element in a larger system—that is to say, it might very well depend for its full effectiveness on the synergistic effect of other substances—and you might have more work than you wanted exploring the biochemics of that larger system. But perhaps overriding even those problems is one that arises from the financial structure of the pharmaceutical industry today. The money behind these companies is in the international banks in Luxembourg and Switzerland. They are not going to spend it in a country that makes it prohibitive to develop a pharmacology—and that's what the United States is these days. Because of the unbelievable tangle of federal regulations and constraints here, the United States takes an excessive amount of time to get therapeutic and curative substances into use, even when they have been used successfully for years in Europe and elsewhere. For example, it has taken us the past ten years to get H2 blocker into the treatment of peptic ulcer, whereas it has been in use in England and continental Europe for ten to fifteen years now. The result of all this is that the United States has ceased to be the real center of pharmacological research. Instead, you're getting reports of advances from places like the United Kingdom, or Argentina, or Mexico.''

Where are we to look for the truth in such a situation? How about in some serious research? Certainly, not a whole lot of that has been done so far. Nobody really knows what B-15 can do for cancer, or for anything else, for that matter. But if it *can* do even a little to help those afflicted by this dread malady, isn't it worth our seeing what, if anything, that might be? Certainly, anybody with an interest in easing suffering and curing disease has no reason to fear such an inquiry. Yet, somehow, we are still waiting.

7

The FDA:
Watchdog or Villain?

No matter which way you turn as you pick your way through the bullets covering the War of B-15, you eventually run into the question of the FDA. What is it *really* doing? Is it merely soldiering on, manfully accomplishing its legally appointed job in protecting the consumer from new, unproven, and possibly dangerous substances? Or is it the tool and stooge of the pharmaceutical, medical, and food processing industries, implacably hostile to anything that might help Americans get well and stay well without resorting to expensive medicines, painful treatments, and heavy doctors' bills?

Depends on who you ask.

Certainly, a lot of people involved with the B-15 controversy who are firmly convinced of B-15's enormous benefit and potential are extremely nervous over the possibility of FDA reprisals if they openly avow their opinions, or if they publicly acknowledge using B-15 in treating their patients. That is why there are so many nameless interviews in this book. For every doctor—or even lay individual—who agrees to let his name be used, there are several others who insist on anonymity. Some clinics require that you disguise their geographical location. Some doctors ask worriedly if you can be forced to reveal your sources and hesitate even to grant anonymous interviews. Scientists experimenting with B-15 under laboratory conditions are apprehensive that their work will be cut off in midstream if the FDA learns who and where they are. So no matter what the FDA's motives and purposes may really be, the *fear* of them is a hard fact in the B-15 debate. It makes for a highly charged emotional atmosphere, to say the least. As one manufacturer, who claims he was verbally abused and threatened by a local FDA official, said, "When someone walks in the door with a loaded revolver and is childlike in his mentality, I guess I stand at attention."

The FDA will tell you that it is merely doing its job. The law is the law, they will say, and they are carrying it out the way they are charged to do. First, they argue, B-15 hasn't got any recognized standard formulation, so the customer doesn't really know what he's getting. Second, it isn't one of the forty some substances appearing on the GRAS—that's "Generally Recognized As Safe"—list appearing in Title 21, Section 121.101, page 315, of the Code of Federal Regulations. That means it's a food additive; because under the Food, Drug, and Cosmetic Act, as amended in 1958, any food product that has not been sold in the United States and was not generally recognized as safe for the purpose intended prior to 1958 is in fact a food additive and must be shown by proper tests to be safe. The burden of proof, moreover, is on the manufacturer. He has to file a food additive petition and prove safety. Nobody has done this with B-15 so far, so the substance is being marketed illegally; and, by law, the FDA is required to put a stop to it.

Representatives of the health food industry greet this argument with scorn. Mere posturing, they say. That's not really why the FDA is out to get B-15. They're just furious because they lost a big one when the Vitamin Bill got through Congress back in 1976. That stopped them from classifying as a "drug" anything over 150 percent of the Recommended Daily Allowance (RDA) of all vitamins and minerals and thus subjecting nearly everything in any health food store to FDA controls. And they really wanted that, because they're in the pocket of the pharmaceutical giants and the medical industry, and if there's one thing those guys hate, it's something that challenges the idea that you always need to go to a doctor to get well. "Promulgation of nutritional concepts—particularly in the form of food supplements—could seriously damage the food and drug businesses," declares Dr. Robert Atkins. "I could 'tranquilize' anyone by using a nutritional program as effectively as by using Valium, which is the largest-selling tranquilizing drug. But that would represent a serious threat to the multibillion-dollar drug industry. And as for the food industry, it has a vested interest in fostering the belief that all you need in your diet are the four basic food groups. So food supplements constitute a threat to it as well."

Needless to say, each side believes firmly that it is in the right, and so the battle goes on, with a court case looming in the very near future. After years of skirmishing, the FDA and the chief manufacturer of B-15, FoodScience/Da Vinci Laboratories, are finally going to court to argue out the matter for good. Although neither side at present is likely to reveal the details of its legal arguments, the proceedings will probably boil down to a struggle over the following contentious questions: first, is B-15 a vitamin, a food, or a food additive; and second, whose responsibility is it to prove the matter one way or the other?

The FDA, of course, adamantly maintains that B-15 is not a vitamin, because nobody has identified a deficiency disease caused by insufficient quantities of it. That puts the FDA on pretty firm ground in declaring that anything labeled "Vitamin B-15" is out of line. B-15 proponents over the years have frequently cited the respected Merck Index as corroboration of their claims that B-15 is indeed a vitamin, because both "B-15" and "pangamic acid" have been listed there since the 1960 edition. But on closer inspection, that turns out to be not quite the sturdy support that some B-15 advocates say it is. When queried on the subject, the editor of the 9th edition said that while both entries would again be included, this didn't mean that B-15 was a vitamin. "It's only to tell the public that the words exist in the chemical literature," she said.

Well, is it a food? FoodScience/Da Vinci Laboratories

insists that it is. "It's a non-fuel nutrient," says Dom Orlandi, "not a vitamin and not a food additive either. It's something the body needs for proper cell chemistry, and it occurs naturally in the body. I can't patent it, because it's a natural substance, and the FDA can't tell me it's a food additive either." If it is a *food,* then the burden of proof is on the *FDA* to show that it is *un*safe, because under the law a simple food need only be reasonably safe to be marketed without FDA supervision. It doesn't even have to be completely safe. Health food advocates are quick to point out that sugar is extremely dangerous to a lot of people, and probably bad for everybody, and except for sheer calories devoid of nutrition. Yet sugar is not only marketed as a food, it is also freely added to other foods. So why the fuss over B-15, they ask?

If it's a food *additive,* the burden of proof is on the *manufacturer* to prove that it's safe. That is a long, hard process, and neither side wants to have to assume responsibility for it. But if B-15 can be designated a food additive, the FDA is in a position of advantage just because it can go on blocking B-15's sale until proof is forthcoming that it is non-toxic.

Actually, the FDA is in a position of advantage right now no matter what the manufacturer does. For example, it can go on impeding B-15's marketing until a manufacturer is forced to ask a court for a declaratory judgment, at which point it is up to the manufacturer to prove that the FDA should back off. Or, the FDA can keep seizing and embargoing B-15 until a harried manufacturer goes to court to get his merchandise back. Again, the FDA will argue that the court should not release the goods because B-15 is not recognized as safe—and the burden of proving it so is again on the manufacturer. Or, finally, an exasperated manufacturer may finally decide he has to go the FDA's route and follow the established procedure for getting an additive approved. Again, it's up to him to prove his case. In fact, even if the manufacturer doesn't go all the way with a food additive petition, and just decides to prove non-toxicity on his own, he is still in effect acknowledging the government's definition of B-15 as a food additive. Once he does that, he has blocked off several possible marketing avenues for himself, because if he makes any health or therapeutic claims for something designated as a food additive, he's sure to run into trouble with some governmental agency, probably the Federal Trade Commission.

It's unlikely in the extreme that the FDA will relent unless it's told to do so by a court of law. Its animus towards B-15 is too entrenched and too longstanding to be dissolved in any other way, from all appearances. But B-15's proponents have some strong, solid arguments, scientific and legal alike, that they can draw on. Moreover, some of them see hope in the fact that a court might be more likely than the FDA to admit that scientific and nutritional research done in other countries—which at present the FDA dismisses out of hand—might just have some validity. Health food industry members point out that our nation's track record in this regard, not to mention the FDA's, has been anything but admirable in recent years.

Meanwhile, no one has ever found B-15 to be harmful. Even the FDA concedes it hasn't received any consumer complaints about it. But that hasn't prevented the FDA from actively obstructing its distribution and sale—sometimes with something that looks enough like vindictiveness for one to understand why many B-15 advocates call it a vendetta. What sometimes seems most galling is the sheer capriciousness of the FDA's behavior. For example, back in 1975, a man in California, Joe De Silva, former head of the 25,000-member Retail Clerks Union, became convinced that certain diseases and metal disorders were the result of biochemical defects that could be nutritionally treated. He had come to this conclusion by a very personal route. In 1968, somebody De Silva cared about had been diagnosed as a hopeless schizophrenic. She had been in and out of hospitals for many months, but no cure was in sight, and the doctors predicted she would become a permanent resident of some mental institution. De Silva would not and could not accept this. So he read every book about schizophrenia he could get this hands on and canvassed all the work that had been done on the subject outside the United States.

And it paid off. De Silva found his solution in large amounts of one particular B vitamin called niacin, or B-3. The niacin transformed the afflicted woman into a normal person who was able to hold a responsible job successfully. In large part as a result of this experience, De Silva subsequently opened his own vitamin and mineral distributing company.

While surveying overseas nutritional research, De Silva had become aware of the impressive amount of foreign data on B-15. So, in November 1975, he went to visit Marvin Taunton, FDA head in Los Angeles, to talk about permission to market B-15 in California. He brought with him a bottle of B-15 (the DMG version) and a report of a safety test performed for FoodScience Labs by Pharmacopathics Research in Maryland—an independent lab which also conducts tests for the FDA—showing that B-15 had been proven safe in experiments on laboratory rats. De Silva knew that if the FDA wanted to ban or suppress something, they had full power to do so, and so he wanted their okay to market the FoodScience product before he accepted any consignment of it.

De Silva showed Taunton the bottle of pills and the safe toxicity report. "I want to know if anything's wrong with the labeling," he said.

Taunton looked at the report and the bottle and gave his okay. "We're not going to touch it," he said.

Then De Silva made his mistake. He didn't get it in writing.

On the strength of Taunton's verbal approval, De Silva ordered $20,000 of B-15 from FoodScience Laboratories. But after he received it, at the end of November, without advance warning or any written legal authority, California Health agents presented themselves at De Silva's warehouse and embargoed the bottles of B-15.

"They looked like a bunch of Keystone Kops with their badges," De Silva relates angrily. He was outraged. He had received the FDA's verbal approval and now, for a reason not given him, the B-15 was being locked up. He knew that even if the FDA never came up with a legal reason, the embargo could still keep the product in limbo for a year until it was considered outdated merchandise and therefore no longer suitable for sale. Heads I win, tails you lose, in effect.

De Silva went back to the FDA to protest the embargo. This time, he spoke to Michael Bogumill, Supervising Food and Drug Specialist, Health Fraud Component of the State of California. The problem, he was told, appeared to be the printing of "B-15" on the label.

"According to the medical authorities upon whom we depend for expert opinion, there is no such thing as Vitamin B-15," Bogumill told him. Several weeks after the embargo, Bogumill wrote De Silva an explanation and authorization for the embargo. First, he wrote, as a dietary supplement B-15 was considered a food additive that had no effective regulation providing for its safe use, and was therefore adulterated. Second, the product was misbranded because the label said it contained a substance, B-15, that was not generally recognized as safe by experts in the field of nutrition. Last, the labeling and advertising material used to promote the product brought it within the definition of a "drug"; and new drugs could not be legally sold to the general public in the state unless there had been prior approval by either the FDA or the Food and Drug Section of the California Department of Health. (This last charge referred to the translated reprints of the Soviet studies made available to health food stores stocking B-15 so that they might be informed of its usages.)

There is, in fact, nothing really wrong with this line of reasoning, if one is thinking solely in terms of enforcing the letter of the existing law to its utmost. And so, one might believe the FDA fully justified—within its own lights, at least—in its opposition to B-15, if it were not for the troubling fact that its zeal seems substantially less when other substances are concerned—notably those representing major established economic interests.

Take, for example, the well-known case of Red Dye #2. For years, Red #2 used to be found in everything from cosmetics to ice cream, despite mounting evidence that it was carcinogenic. Independent testing of this dye on rats had indicated that the animals developed a high incidence of cancerous tumors, and as far back as 1962 there were officials of the National Cancer Institute pointing out that Red #2 was a potential cause of cancer. The FDA's tests, however, proved inconclusive because the rats used in them were accidentally fed incorrect amounts of dye, so that FDA scientists wanted the study invalidated because of the mix-up. This might well have been a perfectly honest mistake, although it still suggests considerable incompetence on the part of the investigators. But those who harbor suspicions of the FDA's good faith point to the fact that Red #2 had been used in more than $10 billion worth of foods each year, and that in 1974 alone the Red #2 industry grossed an estimated $4 million. The FDA now takes credit for having removed Red #2 from the market as a potential risk to public health. But it did take them something like fourteen years to do it, during which time they frequently defended the dye and refused to remove it from the food supply. So it is not altogether surprising that some contrast this with the FDA's zeal over banning B-15 and suggest dubious motives at work.

Then there's the case of another "safe additive," the livestock growth-stimulating hormone, diethylstilbestrol (or "DES"). DES is known to cause cancer, but for many years it has been used to fatten cattle. Indeed, the director of the National Cancer Institute has advised women in their first three months of pregnancy to avoid eating beef liver because it may contain residues of this cancer-causing substance. In 1973, after some ten years of pressure, the FDA finally banned DES, but a U.S. Court of Appeals decision nullified the order a year later saying that the FDA had not given manufacturers a full hearing. Meanwhile, the FDA still approves DES as a "morning-after" birth control pill, despite the fact that DES prescribed to prevent miscarriages in women during the 1950's is now being linked with fatal vaginal and cervical cancer in their grown daughters. If one is so inclined, one can wonder why the FDA finds DES—a known carcinogen—to be acceptable, while B-15—which has no known toxic effects at all—arouses its ire to such a degree.

Some of the stories one comes across while researching this quadrant of the B-15 battlefield are in truth pretty disturbing. There's the story of how, in August 1974, a group of disillusioned FDA employees, including three outside consultants to the Administration, went to Senator Edward Kennedy to air their grievances. "When in the course of their [FDA] duties, they raised questions about new drugs that manufacturers wanted to put on the market, they were frequently overruled by their superiors," wrote Daniel S. Greenberg, an expert in science and government, in the February 1975 issue of *Science Digest*. "When they persisted in expressing doubts about safety and efficacy, they were often reprimanded, denied promotion, and in some cases transferred to 'make-work' jobs or duties that were unrelated to their training and experience."

Greenberg continued, "No such flaps, however, arose when they approved applications for new drugs. In such cases, the approvals whizzed through the bureaucratic process without question." Senator Kennedy was to say after the Congressional Committee heard the FDA employees' complaints: "The testimony of all these witnesses was strikingly similar and very disheartening."

Then there's the story of how an antibiotic drug called Chloramphenicol, manufactured by Parke-Davis, was held responsible shortly after its release for destruction of blood cells, causing several deaths from anemia. Dr. Joseph F. Sadusk, Director of the FDA Bureau of Medicine at the time, could have withdrawn it from the market. Instead, he seems to have prevented the drug from being recalled and apparently even ruled against requiring a precautionary label. In time Chloramphenicol was replaced by a newer product, and Parke-Davis, its manufacturer, sent a letter to all physicians stating that it was no longer the drug of choice for any of the infections it originally had been designed to cure. At no point was any mention made of its damaging effects. A short time later, Sadusk left the FDA and, within the year, accepted a new job—as vice-president of Parke-Davis.

Nor is this the only instance in which FDA officials have subsequently taken jobs with the companies they were charged with regulating. In 1961, Peter Hutt left his post as Chief Attorney for Food Processing Companies to become FDA Legal Counsel. Simultaneously, William Goodrich, the outgoing FDA Counsel, took Peter Hutt's old job. At other times, a former Deputy FDA Commissioner went to the conglomerate representing a well-advertised peanut butter and mayonnaise, and an FDA Director for the Office of Product Technology left to take a post with a canned goods corporation. None of this can be called clear evidence of illicit dealings. It is more or less inevitable that people will move on from their present jobs to jobs with people they have worked with, who know them and who value their abilities. But it is hard to escape the impression of at times closer affinity of interests than one might wish between the FDA and the giant industries it is charged with policing.

It is these suspicions that make some people wonder if the FDA is acting in good faith in the matter of B-15. Given the known and seemingly rather numerous instances in the past in which the FDA has looked with complaisance upon the marketing of substances whose health hazards were known, why does it rise up in its wrath to protect the public against something that even it concedes has never hurt anybody? The FDA reply to that argument is that nobody has proven that the substance won't hurt anybody—but if that is so, why has the FDA in the past delayed so long, years in fact, before banning substances that *were* known to hurt somebody? Somehow, one begins to feel, you can't have it both ways.

The health food industry is firmly convinced that the FDA is out to get it, and to support their claim they cite instances of what they call FDA harassment. B-15's proponents have a lot of war stories like that; and, in point of fact, some of them do sound very much indeed like harassment. For example, in 1978 FDA attorney Ronald Craig telephoned a famous West

Coast university, one of whose professors, who holds both an M.D. and a Ph.D. in biochemistry, has been doing controlled experiments in cooperation with FoodScience/Da Vinci Laboratories, to assess the effect of B-15, in the form of N,N-Dimethylglycine, on laboratory animals. (The professor will probably also serve as a witness for FoodScience in the upcoming court case.) Craig informed the professor's department head that if the professor continued with this "testimony in favor of those crooks," as he described the owners of FoodScience/Da Vinci, the FDA would ruin the university's reputation as well as the professor's. The department head's note informing the professor of this telephone conversation is now in the hands of FoodScience's attorneys.

Sometimes the stories sound less like harassment than petty spite. For example, one of FoodScience's young salesmen remarks that he is aware that several of the firm's telephone lines are tapped by the FDA. "Many times when I talk to a doctor," he says, "I realize that I'm talking over a tapped line. So I always say to him, 'Doctor, I'm going to tell you how to treat your patients with a certain nutritional product. But, of course, you realize that this means I am practising medicine without a license, and that the FDA is listening. So before I go any further, let me just say that if the FDA is interested, my home address is . . . and my telephone number is . . .' I do this in a very joking manner, of course, but that's what's going on. And it's not just us. A lot of the doctors in practice, who use and believe in nutrition as a preventive and curative tool, are repeatedly harassed by the FDA."

Sometimes, the stories can sound as much like incompetence as malice—a confusion familiar enough to anybody who has worked closely with the government. Take the story of how the FDA blundered its way through a seizure-and-embargo action in the Midwest. Some time ago, a truckload of B-15 was on its way from a factory in the Midwest to a distributor in the East. When it had gotten about 20 miles from the factory—long before it had crossed any state line—six state patrol cars materialized from the roadside, red lights flashing. In them, along with a number of state police officers, were two federal FDA agents and two men from the State Department of Agriculture. They asked permission to get into the truck. The driver refused. They went in anyway, although that commonly requires a search warrant. Picking out a bottle of the B-15, the FDA agent said, "This is what we're after." Then the whole caravan returned to the factory. After a pointed exchange with the factory owner, the FDA agents departed, leaving one man from the State Department of Agriculture behind, and saying that they were going to embargo the B-15 under a state law that embargoes any food product which is adulterated or misbranded.

Predictably, however, the factory owner was thoroughly familiar with that law. This wasn't his first skirmish with the FDA. He knew that in the first paragraph of the necessary embargo forms, it said that the State agent must have had prior knowledge of what was in the truck and prior knowledge that it was misbranded or adulterated. So he asked the State Agriculture inspector if he had ever been in this factory, and if he knew the factory owner. The inspector replied, no, he was ordinarily a milk inspector, this was something new for him. This meant the FDA was sending someone to embargo a product who didn't know what the product was—and that, under the law, amounted to conspiracy. The factory owner then wrote across the embargo forms that the inspector didn't know the product and had never been in the building, and the inspector signed it.

Next, the owner filed suit against the federal government, the state government, and the individual inspector. The FDA prepared its case poorly; indeed, the owner thinks they made several technical errors purposely because they really didn't want it to go to court. So the factory owner wound up winning the case by default. He could then have sued the FDA for loss of property, but as he said, the property never actually got lost so he really didn't have grounds for that.

This same factory owner goes on to relate that for the past three or four years, every time the FDA inspectors came in with questions about B-15, he would say, yes, he made it and would then ask each individual inspector in turn if there was something wrong with that. Invariably, he says, they would say, no, they were just checking. Fine, he would say, because if there's something wrong with it, send me an affidavit and I won't make it. "I must have done that ten times over a period of three years," he notes with satisfaction, "and every time, they said there's nothing wrong with it. Of course, they don't sign affidavits—I know that—but you have to put them on the spot, and it's nice to ask them and have them not do it!"

Inconsistency, malice, incompetence, or maybe just plain confusion? You can put whatever interpretation you want on these stories and come up with your own assessment of the FDA's real role in the B-15 battle. But for me the quintessential story, however, a tale that captures all the lingering air of double-think hanging over the FDA's record in banning or releasing one thing or another, is the story—the *true* story!—that I call "The FDA and the Plain Brown Wrapper."

It seems that there was a doctor in the Midwest who was acquainted with a District Commissioner of the FDA. One day, the Commissioner called him up and told him that the FDA was going to take B-15 off the market.

"Don't do that!" cried the doctor. "We need it for our athletes!" (The doctor does a lot of work with young athletes training for competitions.)

"Don't be silly," retorted the Commissioner. "That stuff doesn't work."

Then, a few weeks later, the Commissioner calls up again. He's feeling awfully tired these days, he says, and he wonders if the doctor could recommend something to help him.

"But don't send me any of that B-15," he warned, "because I know it doesn't work."

The doctor didn't say anything. He just sent the Commissioner a supply of pills in a plain brown bottle, labeled something noncommittal like "supervitamin," and waited to see what happened. The pills, however, were N,N-Dimethylglycine. Good old B-15.

A couple of weeks later, sure enough, the telephone rings, and it's the Commissioner. "Whatever that stuff is that you gave me, it's gotten me feeling great," he raved. "As a matter of fact, I wonder if you could send some of the same stuff to one of the Commissioners in Washington, D.C., in the Medical Division Department."

"Do you know what you've been taking?" inquired the doctor.

"No."

"You've been taking B-15," the doctor told him.

A brief silence ensued. "You've got to be kidding," the Commissioner finally replied, "but I don't really care what it is, it works. Can you send some to my boss in Washington?"

The doctor agreed, and once again he put the little white pills in a plain brown bottle, labeled it "supervitamin," and sent it off.

About ten days later, the Washington official calls up and says, "Hey, I'm doing great. Send me some more of that supervitamin stuff!"

"Do you know what that 'supervitamin stuff' is?" the doctor asked again.

"No, why?"

"That's B-15."

Another silence.

"Well," came the response at last, "I still want you to send me some more—but please, don't label it!"

Where To
From Here?

Where does this all leave us? We've heard some people rave
about B-15 while others declare it a ripoff. We've heard some
medical practitioners insist that B-15 yields excellent results in
their practice, while others, equally qualified and sincere, de-
bunk it as worthless. Every report of a dramatic benefit seems
to raise more questions than it answers. At the same time,
every denunciation of B-15 requires an act of selective inat-
tention whereby some very intriguing, even if inconclusive,
evidence is deliberately ignored.

A lot is at stake. *If* B-15 can do even a fraction of the
things that some of its advocates think it can, it could be a
phenomenal addition to the tools of medical science. And if it
can do *any* of these things, and we dismiss it before we know
for sure, with no effort to explore its potential, we have in
effect cheated ourselves. On the other hand, if dispassionate
inquiry reveals that B-15 is in fact overrated, we will at least
know for sure and can put the dream to rest.

We need more research on two major fronts. First, we need
to establish the proper chemical formulation of the substance
called B-15 and then learn what actually happens in the internal chemistry of the cell when that substance is introduced into
the body system. Second, we need more rigorously designed
clinical experiments under controlled conditions to establish

B-15's effects on disease. As part of this effort, we need to explore the question of synergism—that is, the question of whether B-15 works better (assuming that it works at all) in association with other substances such as vitamins and minerals, and if so, which ones and in what amounts.

In fact, some researchers have already begun to experiment along these lines, and the results of their studies, when they become fully available in the next year or so, should begin to fill this crippling information vacuum that now distorts the B-15 debate. These researchers have insisted upon complete anonymity here, because they are extremely anxious that the FDA not descend upon them until their results can be analyzed and published in reputable medical journals. So the names associated with the experiments described hereafter are disguised, and in some cases even their geographical location is changed. The experiments, however, are real, and their outcome may prove very important to the health of us all.

Dr. Ari Purchase, a California cardiovascular specialist who also holds a Ph.D. in biochemistry, began using B-15 (in the form of N,N-Dimethylglycine) two years ago with his heart patients. So many of these told him that they felt better on B-15 that he decided to look into its effects more systematically. Besides which, he had been reading the Soviet reports and had concluded that the Russians were exaggerating. He decided something better was needed, so he designed a study using over 100 volunteer patients from his own large practice. Half of these were suffering from angina pectoris, the chest pain that afflicts many heart sufferers. About a fifth of them were hypertensive, with seriously high blood pressure. About a third had circulatory inhibitions due to the slowness with which their impaired hearts pumped blood through their bodies. All were given three tablets of DMG per day—a modest dosage since most people take six tablets per day. All the patients were tested for cholesterol levels, triglycerides (that is, the fat content in the blood), blood flow rates, and blood pressure at the beginning of the experiment, at six months, and again at eleven months.

The results were striking. At the beginning of the study, all the angina pectoris sufferers were on drugs to relieve their pain. After six months, half of these were able to give up all drugs. At the eleven-month mark, two thirds were off all drugs. All said they felt better and had less pain, and they seemed to walk and move with less effort.

Of those patients with high blood pressure, more than a third were off drugs after six months, while two thirds were able to do without drugs after eleven months. Nearly half of those with circulatory inhibitions showed improvement by the end of the study period.

Cholesterol and triglyceride levels showed significant drops. In the beginning, the cholesterol level ranged from 300–400 mg percent for the whole group of subjects. After six months, 40 percent of them had dropped to 290 mg percent. After eleven months, nearly half had dropped to 210 mg percent. At the study's inception, triglyceride levels ranged from 225–400 mg percent. After six months, 40 percent of all subjects had an average level of 180 mg percent, and after eleven months, this average was down to 140 mg percent.

How much of this could be due to the placebo effect? After all, these people had volunteered for this experiment and one would presume that they had done so in the hope that they would feel better as a result. If only subjective evidence had been forthcoming—if they had only reported that they *felt* better or that it *seemed* that they could move with more ease—one might discount the results on those grounds. But the presence of objective as well as subjective results means that something was really happening to their body systems. The group's blood pressure fell significantly. Their vascular tone—that is, the rate of blood flow through their veins and arteries—improved. Their cholesterol and triglyceride levels dropped. Their electrocardiograms showed better T-wave characteristics and progress in eliminating arrhythmias, or irregularities in the heartbeat.

Dr. Purchase also undertook to explore the matter of synergism in this experiment. Along with the group given

B-15 alone, another group of equal size was given the same amount of B-15, that is, three tablets a day, plus 400–800 units each of selenium, silicon, and mixed tocopherols. The results showed that this group did a little better than the one given B-15 alone. They felt a little better, had more energy and better exercise tolerance. Their triglycerides and cholesterol were somewhat lower, and their blood pressure came down somewhat more.

Well, Dr. Purchase is asked, does he think B-15 produced the good results he got? "All I know is what my tests showed," he responds cautiously. "People on B-15 told me they felt better, and my tests showed objective improvements in blood flow, blood pressure, circulatory inhibitions, triglycerides, and cholesterol. I don't know if it was B-15 that actually *caused* these changes, but that's what happened.

"I'm trying to establish a modicum of preventive medicine in the profession," Dr. Purchase goes on. "It's time we got some of these people and kept them from becoming cardiovascular. It's high time we started with a *younger* group and worked to *keep* them from reaching the sort of state they are usually in when they come for treatment. This may be greeted with considerable hostility in the medical profession, of course, because it digs into the pocketbook if people are not getting sick so badly so often. Also, the pharmaceutical houses are likely to balk. But somebody's got to do it."

Dr. Purchase's results find reinforcement in those obtained by another experimenter, Dr. Peter Sebastian, a scientist working in the Midwest. (Again, remember that these are fictitious names to protect these scientists from premature exposure. But the experiments and their results are real.) Dr. Sebastian became interested in B-15 (in the form of DMG) about a year ago, when he was treating a group of diabetics, all of whom were overweight and had circulatory problems. The most dramatic case was that of a diabetic amputee. She had already lost one leg and was having circulatory problems in the other one, which was strongly cyanotic, very cold and painful. Her cholesterol was above 300, and her triglycerides were over

500, which was off the chart. Her alkaline phosphotese (liver fraction) was also elevated. After 20 days on DMG, her cholesterol was within normal limits, her triglycerides had fallen to 374, and her alkaline phosphotese had dropped from 128 to 109.

These remarkable results led Dr. Sebastian to investigate what effects DMG might have on patients with heart problems. His preliminary experimental group consists of slightly more than 50 patients with heart problems. "We start with fasting, a diagnostic profile over thirteen tests, including the serum tests as well as the differentials, and then urinalysis. We do the blood tests at zero, ten, thirty, and sixty days. We also do pulse volume or Doppler ultrasound recordings, or both, of the upper and lower extremities on a vascular diagnostic analyzer. That's a machine that does a graph of the extremities, both arterial and venous, to see if we have any changes in the blood flow rate.

"All the patients were put on 100 mg of dimethylglycine hydrochloride per day. We are definitely seeing change in the serum lipids.[1] With patients having very high serum lipids the first change we see is an immediate reduction in cholesterol, triglycerides, and the different groups within the triglyceride lipoproteins. In patients where the serum lipids are medium high, we usually see an increase during the first ten days, followed by a continual decrease over a period of sixty days. To date, I have not seen a single case that had elevated serum lipids where we have not seen a decrease in their level over a period of sixty days.

"We had one coronary patient who had been documented as having triglycerides over 400 now for four years, with no response to chemotherapy. After ninety days on di-methylglycine hydrochloride, the triglycerides and the

---

[1]*Lipid:* any one of a group of fats and fat-like substances having in common the property of insolubility in water and solubility in fat solvents. Included are fats, fatty acids, fatty oils, waxes, sterols, and esters of fatty acids containing other groups such as phosphoric acid (phospholipids) and carbohydrates (glycolipids).

cholesterol in this patient dropped to normal levels, whereas previously they had been sky-high."

When this preliminary experiment is completed, Dr. Sebastian plans to embark upon a full-scale, crossover double-blind experiment involving 200 patients, 100 of which will be on DMG hydrochloride and the other 100 on a placebo. The 100 on the placebo will then be cross-matched and put on the DMG. The end result will be 200 patients who have been on DMG. Dr. Sebastian has already begun the experiment, as of this writing, and the results, when available, should be as unassailable as such things can be, inasmuch as his experimental design is as rigorous as possible. When interviewed, Dr. Sebastian stated that the preliminary study's results were very encouraging.

Further research is also in progress relative to B-15's effect on the immune response, that mechanism in the bloodstream that mobilizes the body's defenses against infection and disease. Dr. Miles Champion has been investigating this in his work at a major medical school in the Southeast. "We looked into it because somebody had said the Russians had found that calcium pangamate was an immuno-adjuvant, that is, something that when used along with some immunogen causes heightened immune response. Well, as it turned out, we never found anything about that in the Russian literature, but we still wanted to look into it, because it is such an important area.

"We got some B-15 from Da Vinci Laboratories, and decided to test it out on laboratory rabbits. We used a test group of six animals and a control group of the same number. All twelve were given typhoid antigens, and the test group was given the B-15. Then we bled them at two-week intervals over a period of six weeks and analyzed the blood. We found that the test group had a statistically significant humoral immune response—in other words, there was a significant increase in antibodies in the test group over the control group.

"I've hesitated to publish this study, however, because I'm not sure we used the optimal dosage of B-15. In theory, you might calibrate the dose proportionally to the body weight of your laboratory animals relative to that of a human. But after kicking it around for a while, we settled on a much larger dose that would equate to quite a massive dose in a human. It certainly didn't hurt the rabbits. But I think we need to run the experiment again using smaller doses and determine what the optimal one would be."

Meanwhile, some of Dr. Champion's colleagues tried DMG on blood samples from a small group of humans, of whom some were normal, some were diabetic, and some had sickle cell anemia. The group was quite small, and consequently the results are only preliminary. But the experimenters found them encouraging. They conveyed their findings in a letter that requires extensive translation of its technical language before a layperson can make head or tail of it. They began by giving some background: "In 1960," they write, "P. C. Nowell discovered that phytohemagglutinin (PHA), a lectin [first translation: a lectin is a plant product that has the property of agglutinating red blood cells] extracted from kidney beans, could cause the transformation of lymphocytes in tissue culture into proliferating lymphoblasts." Time out for further translation: lymphocytes are a type of white blood cell that accounts for about 40 percent of your white blood cell population. In the presence of a "mitogen," i.e., something that triggers the blood's reaction to infection, healthy lymphocytes will start multiplying dramatically, at something like thirty times their normal rate. But *un*healthy lymphocytes, such as those from people with diabetes or sickle cell anemia, will hardly react at all, dividing once or twice instead of thirty times. A lymphocyte that is in the process of becoming two lymphocytes during this multiplication process is called a "lymphoblast," and the process itself is called "lymphocyte blast transformation," or "LBT."

Therefore, what the letter is saying is that adding PHA to blood would make lymphocytes start multiplying, setting in motion a series of further reactions that would ultimately allow the body to neutralize infection. Got it? Okay, the letter goes on: "Since that time, LBT [that is, lymphocyte blast transformation] has been regarded as a classic in vitro measure of in vivo cell-mediated immune responsiveness.'' What this means is that this process wherein lymphocytes start multiplying madly is an accepted yardstick for measuring in a test tube (''in vitro'') the effectiveness with which the immune response is proceeding in the living body (''in vivo'').

Still there? What all this leads up to, finally, is the statement that ''DMG definitely has an 'enhancing' effect on LBT in patient and normal populations.'' In plain English, DMG makes the immune response work better in both sick people and normal people.

Attached to the letter were some preliminary bar charts showing the results of blood tests taken before and after adding DMG to blood samples from normal persons, diabetics, and some with sickle cell anemia. In each case, the tests improved after adding the DMG, which seemed to normalize lymphocytes from diabetics and ''sicklers'' so that they began multiplying at a better rate, one closer to that of normal lymphocytes.

The letter concluded that the explanation of all this is lacking and that ''we have a long way to go before DMG has good credibility . . . [but] I feel the data shows promise of elucidating some of DMG's beneficial effects.''

Another West Coast researcher, Dr. Reinhold Kreisky, who also holds an M.D. and a Ph.D. in biochemistry, has done work involving DMG's effects on stress and hypoxia (oxygen starvation). ''I found that dimethylglycine definitely lowers the lactic acid level in the blood serum of stressed animals,'' he reports. ''I anesthetized a group of rabbits. Then I attached their veins and arteries to transducers that measured the blood pressure in those blood vessels. Their breathing was controlled by a special engine to which their trachea were directly connected. The rabbits were not in pain, because of the anesthesia, but the preparations were a great stress to them. Then I monitored the level of carbon dioxide in the blood, and every three to four hours I took a blood sample and measured the lactic acid levels. The group that had been given DMG had well-balanced breathing, and their lactic acid levels were much lower than the control group, subjected to the same stress, but not given DMG."

Remember that lactic acid build-up is directly associated with fatigue. Dr. Kreisky's results corroborate the claim that B-15 (at least in the form of DMG, which was the version he used) can increase stamina by holding down lactic acid levels.

Dr. Kreisky also explored DMG's potential for improving oxygen utilization. "I took a group of rats," he begins, "and I put each one into a special cage that had a measuring device to measure the oxygen in the air. I started with about 21 percent oxygen content, which is the equivalent of sea level. Then I let the oxygen level drop to 17 percent, which equates to an altitude of about 4–5,000 feet. Then I went to 13 percent, which equates to an altitude of about 10,000 feet and brings on hypoxia. I found that the rats treated with DMG could use oxygen in the same way at the 13 percent oxygen level as they could in a normal oxygen environment."

Dr. Kreisky's findings corroborate another claim made for B-15, namely, that it increases available oxygen. How many other claims, one wonders, might be similarly substantiated if the necessary experimentation were permitted?

Even when B-15's abilities are properly mapped by experiments such as these, however, we'll need to explore a whole crowd of other questions arising from the characteristically mulish nature of the individual metabolism. It seems that no matter *what* you think a particular substance or nutrient will do, somebody's metabolism is going to surprise you with an unexpected reaction. The results can sometimes be pretty bewildering, and this may well play a part in the wide divergence of results, ranging from marvelous to ho-hum, that B-15 users have reported. One Virginia M.D. who has worked intensively in preventive medicine for years tells how his experience has taught him to expect the unexpected.

"No matter how well documented you think a dietary supplement's effects may be," he notes somewhat ruefully, "there's going to be some patient who will have you scratching your head because his body does something different from what you thought it would. Customarily, for example, a thyroid supplement will 'jazz you up,' sometimes pretty dramatically. But I just had a patient telephone me and complain that the thyroid I had told her to take was making her *sleepy!* Somebody have mercy on the poor prescribing physician!

"Sometimes your problem is that the patient's digestive tract is so badly impaired and so enzyme-depleted that no matter *what* you're giving them, they can't absorb it. As a result of a lifetime of eating low-fiber, highly processed foods and large quantities of milk, the interior walls of the intestine are simply too heavily coated with mucus to let anything get through and be assimilated. Therefore, these people may show *no* effects, good *or* bad, from taking a supplement, even when you raise the dosage to very high levels. And they won't until you get their digestive tract cleaned out so it can begin to do its job again.

"Then there's the problem of proper dosage. The established Minimum Daily Requirements are largely useless as a guide. They will do as a *minimum,* but they may very well be grossly inadequate for some people. To cite only one example, stress can cause vitamin requirements for some people to jump sharply. So your problem is to find out what dosage your patient *does* need, and there's nothing much to help you there except trial and error. For example, I had a woman in here with chronic sinus. I put her on 1500 mg of Vitamin C a day, but after two weeks it hadn't done any good at all. After four weeks without success, I upped the dose to 3000 mg—and her sinus disappeared. Yet 1500 mg is a fairly hefty dosage for most people.

"Then there was a man with a bad prostate problem. I put him on the 'normal' dosage of zinc, i.e., 15 mg a day. Nothing happened. Then I tripled the dose and it worked. Another woman had a lot of lower back pain. Medication hadn't helped her. I put her on a calcium supplement, but it didn't help much. Tripling the dose, on the other hand, did the trick. Yet on all her heart and blood tests her calcium levels had shown up normal!

"As if this weren't enough, you also have the problem of hidden allergies. Most of these are caused by foods. You can eliminate from the patient's diet all the things you know he is allergic to, but you may find later that he is allergic to things neither of you knew about. For example, some patients get an allergic reaction to some nutrient or supplement you are giving them, and it turns out that they aren't allergic to the substance itself but rather to the *base* in which it is compounded. An example is Vitamin C, which usually comes from corn. If your patient turns out to be allergic to corn, you may have to experiment with several different brands of C before you find one that he can ingest comfortably.

"What it adds up to is that B-15 may be an enormously valuable supplement, but anybody who expects it to do the *same* thing for everyone who takes it is simply naive. It doesn't work that way. You have to work with the idiosyncracies of the patient's own body, and at times it takes skill and inspiration to hit on the right combination of helpful agents."

This physician's observations are enormously provocative for the light they seem to throw on that troubling question: Why do B-15 users report such wildly divergent results? We've already seen that the chemical composition of the "real" B-15 is a confused enough issue for it to be possible that some of those people weren't really taking B-15 at all, regardless of what the label on the bottle might have read. Now comes the possibility that some people's digestive tracts assimilate nutrients so poorly that whatever they might have been taking may never have gotten through their intestinal walls—being excreted instead without having done anything useful along the way. Another possibility we now can see is that some people's requirements might have been far higher than the "normal" dosage—so that where some people might have gotten fantastic results on three tablets a day, somebody else may have needed eight or perhaps ten, and because this didn't occur to them, they didn't get the results they were looking for.

What it all leaves us with is questions. Not a whole lot of answers, but certainly a lot of questions. Questions, moreover, that seem worth taking the gamble to explore, because if it turns out that B-15 can do even *some* of the wonderful things that have been credited to it, it will be a blessing of immense proportions to us all.

And, of course, it all depends on research. Which is exactly what we have too little of right now. Moreover, the situation is likely to stay that way for the indefinite future so long as the seemingly implacable hostility of the medical establishment and the United States government *prevents* such research. A sorry state of affairs indeed . . . especially for a nation that has historically prided itself on its unbounded scientific curiosity and eagerness to probe any scientific puzzle to its depths.

Why such hostility? That was the question that kept bothering me as I researched this book. Ordinarily, one would expect that reports of such astonishing possibilities as have piled up for B-15 would attract eager attention. Yet here one finds an altogether striking unwillingness *even to consider the evidence,* and, instead, an a priori negative reaction that strikes the ear as somehow disproportionately emotional in what is, in theory at least, a factual scientific debate.

I began hearing echoes. The Ptolemaic astronomers furiously denouncing Galileo. The nineteenth century conservative biological establishment decrying Darwin. Traditional medicine ridiculing the theories of Lister and Semmelweiss on germs and surgical antisepsis. In each case, the hostility these men elicited stemmed not from the evidence they had discovered, but from the fact that they were *challengers of basic concepts* about science and medicine. Galileo denied the very foundation upon which not only medieval science but also Catholic theology was erected, namely, the idea that the earth was the center of creation. No, said Galileo. Look at these observations. The planets *can't* move that way if they are circling the earth. Not only was his evidence ignored, he was forced to recant under threat of excommunication. Nobody bothered to consider his evidence on its merits because *that was not what was at issue.* What was at issue were deeply held concepts about the nature of the world and reality, and people change those only under the most strenuous protest.

Similarly, Darwin too was denounced on religious rather than scientific grounds. The staggering amount of data he had collected on his travels around the world was something to be suppressed rather than explored for those who held that the Bible told the story of creation in literal terms. Darwin's theory of evolution thereby became more than a new possible explanation of observable fact; it became instead a challenge to religious conviction, and hence sacrilegious.

Well, religions come in all shapes and sizes, and our supposedly secular age has produced some pretty good examples of the genre, albeit under some odd labels. Marxism, for example, or any deeply revolutionary creed that can make human beings fight and die over political abstractions—these are religions under a different name. And what makes them revolutionary is that they challenge *other* deeply held convictions about the proper nature of the world, not to mention those whose material welfare is rationalized and justified by the older world view.

Science is no exception. Scientific revolutions bear fascinating similarities to political revolutions. In each case, you will find the early rebel, the one who refuses to accept the prevalent ideas about how the world is or ought to be organized. Time and again, this individual is roundly denounced, often persecuted, and more often than not his evidence is simply ignored. Then his idea begins to spread. Evidence accumulates to corroborate his theories, and, finally, enough people have come to believe them to challenge the establishment. Predictably, the establishment resists this challenge to its position, status, and authority, not to mention the material wealth that accrues to it from that authority and position. After some period of intense struggle, the new view triumphs.

And then, yesterday's scientific heresy becomes today's commonplace, and future generations look back and wonder how anyone could have been so stubborn or blind as to think it anything but obvious!

Something of this sort seems to be percolating today in the whole area of medicine and biology—a revolution in thought pivoting on the question of the nature, provenance, and proper treatment of disease. Orthodox medicine was founded upon the concept of disease as an invader from without, an alien intruder into the body mechanism, which may best be eliminated by treatment with counteracting agents such as drugs or surgery. But a rival view is gaining widening adherence now. It regards disease not as something invariably caused by external agents but rather as a creation of the body's own internal disorder. Such a view leads to the further deduction that the best treatment for many diseases is to restore the body's own health-producing mechanisms—with a very heavy emphasis on preventive measures to preclude the disease's eruption in the first place.

Now, this is a proposition that is inevitably going to mobilize powerful resistance from those who have vested interests, economic and emotional alike, in the established medical outlook. And it is against this background that the heated controversy over B-15, otherwise so seemingly unreasonable at times, begins to make sense. If B-15 were just another vitamin or nutrient, it might be pretty hard to explain the level of emotion it elicits. But it is a very great deal more than that. It represents a sizable opening skirmish in what may shape up to be a scientific battle royal that may last the rest of this century, and end by revising our entire notions of medicine and biology.

Biology, some prominent physicians now say, is *not* a science in the proper sense of that word, despite the proud claims made for it. "It's no more than a series of observed phenomena," states Dr. Gary Gordon of the Academy of

American Preventics in Sacramento, "in which we try to say we believe that something like cholesterol, for example, is a risk factor. But it's not at all rigorous in the way that physics or chemistry is. It has no body of established fundamental principles such as Newton's Laws or the Laws of Thermodynamics. Only now is the necessary work being done to give biology this sort of scientific rigor, and it's being done by one of the most brilliant physicians I know, a man who has retired from his practice to devote his full time to this work. He's applying to biology the full panoply of scientific knowledge and principles that we have developed in other fields, such as quantum physics and the principle of uncertainty, and when he gets finished, I think the face of biology as we now know it will be changed forever.

"This man is doing trailblazing work in biological theory, and some of his research is beginning to indicate that B-15 does in fact exist and that it will be found to have the characteristics ascribed to it, and that something like it is certainly going to be needed for proper health. It's a bit like the way in which the existence of the planet Pluto was predicted before anybody had ever sighted it in a telescope. What we had already learned about the solar system told us that there *had* to be another planet out there . . . and, sure enough, when we went looking for it, there it was. Well, I think that's going to be the case with B-15 too."

If, of course, we go looking. Otherwise, we'll never know, one way or the other.